MW00713558

Save the First Dance for You

Dear Reader,

Can the caring profession learn to care for themselves? Can a nurse be the nurse doctor? Are nurses ready to become more self-nurturing and introspective as they care for the needs of the sick and infirm?

We all know that nurses have a stressful job and a caring spirit. The question is: how do these two qualities work for and against them as individuals and as a professional? In this time of nursing shortage, it seems imperative that nurses care for themselves in order to take care of others. In this, her first book, Doris Young achieves her mission to care for the caregiver.

As you will soon see, Young has seen and experienced the way stress bends and sometimes breaks nurses. Her nurturing, empowering words will help nurses achieve their full potential, personally and professionally.

Young's voice is wonderfully engaging yet authoritative. She shares stories from her vast experience of more than 30 years in the field of nursing. The addition of nurses' stories and in-text examples are touching, moving, and inspiring. Her work as a coach and coach trainer brings richness to this terrific source for growth and healing for the nursing profession. Each time that I prepared to add a note about "don't forget your audience," — BAM! — She'd come up with something that spoke to nurses.

Doris Young has done a GREAT job here! It spoke to me more than I can tell you. When it's published, I will be giving copies to my friends.

I do hope she'll consider marketing this beyond nurses in a more general *Save the First Dance For You* down the road. The way she addresses the issues we all face as people is so inviting that it merits very serious consideration by inspirational publishers in the future if Doris chooses to take that step.

So far, editing *Save the First Dance For You* has been one of the most joyful experiences in my twenty-year career. I hope you're ready to join me in bringing the marvelous work to the world of nurses.

—Best wishes,
Melanie Rigney

Save the First Dance for You is an exciting, foundational work that should be required reading for all nurses, from students to retirees. I believe that Dr. Young's wisdom from the heart holds the promise of preventing burnout and transforming the lives of nurses who apply its message. It may even be the catalyst that is needed to revitalize the profession. Wholistic self-care will help us provide better care of the body, mind, and spirit for our patients and loved ones.

—Pamela Larsen Schroeder, MSN, RN,C, CHPN

We have a responsibility to our patients—and to ourselves as well, and that's no joke! In *Save the First Dance for You,* Doris Young gives you the steps to bring your authentic self to your work and prevent burnout.

—Karyn Buxman, RN, MSN, CSP, CPAE
CEO, HUMORx.com

Nurses are in the position of perpetual caring and giving of themselves. Young provides nurses with an important holistic prescription to protect and heal themselves from the spiritual depletion that can result. *Save the First Dance For You* is a wonderful journey back to the authentic self.

Thanks for this important work and for providing me the opportunity to participate.

—Teresa Haller, MSN, MBA, RN
President, Virginia Nurses Association

Doris Young has given nurses a tremendous gift in her book, *Save the First Dance for You*. Her message resonated in my heart and soul because I took ballet and tap at the young age of 8 years old. I have been dancing my way though life always thinking of others and very little of myself. Now that I am a nurse of many years and with great wisdom, I plan to subscribe to the lessons Doris has given me. I started with tears in the first chapter and have finished with renewed spirit and direction. Doris, your book has truly warmed my heart and renewed my spirit. Every nurse should have a copy whether old or young.

—Shirley Tate Gibson
—President, Virginia Organization of Nurse Executives

Save the First Dance for You is a how-to manual nurses can use to prevent and cure burnout, helping their patients by helping themselves. Doris Young encourages us to look at the bigger picture of our lives, to climb up from the bottom of Maslow's pyramid and aim for the top level of self-actualization. In this voyage, we must determine which of our current thinking and behavior patterns hold us back and which move us forward. We learn to assert control over our own lives, instead of simply accepting whatever positions others place us in, especially when they conflict with our own values and principles.

Doris Young explores the "nursing personality" that so many of us share. She shows that many nurses emerge from social backgrounds in which pleasing others seems to be the only way to earn respect and gain self-esteem. After giving much and getting little in return from family, employers, patients, friends or lovers, we may get angry, snap at those who take us for granted, and make harsh demands about what we need for self-preservation. This can confuse and drive away others as it leaves us bitter and unsatisfied.

But *Save the First Dance for You* teaches us how to figure out what we need and seek it in more constructive ways before we get used and abused, helping us achieve more positive human relationships, gratifying careers and ultimately healthier patients.

Under Doris Young's coaching, I can imagine a whole new nursing profession. I see a profession in which nurses are better able to work for: safe patient loads; systemic changes to eliminate dangerous patient care practices, workplaces that value nursing input; nursing-led hospitals and institutions; adequate funding for nursing education, research and clinical practice; insurance reimbursement specifically for nursing care; professional pride; and broad public and media recognition of nurses' true value and health expertise, the lack of which has contributed greatly to the critical underfunding of nursing and the global shortage.

At first, *Save the First Dance for You* may seem like a fantasy to nurses wondering if they will even get a bathroom break on their next 12-hour shift. But those are the nurses who need this book the most. The book can serve as a wonderful tool to help us find the strength in each of us and use it to empower ourselves and our profession. Nurses and our patients need the help that Doris Young's important book is offering us.

—Sandy Summers, RN, MSN, MPH,
Executive Director, Center for Nursing Advocacy

To receive your free gift worth $29 go to
http://www.SavetheFirstDanceforYou.com/relaxation.htm

Save
the First Dance
for You

The Complete Nurse's Guide to
Serving Your Profession, Your
Patients, and YOURSELF

Doris Young, PhD, RN

YOUNG PUBLICATIONS
NORFOLK, VIRGINIA

To my husband,
Michael,
without whom I would not be a dancer
and living a life I love;

and to my son,
Matthew,
the most incredible young man I know
who fills my life with the greatest joy;

and to my mother,
Mary Doris,
my first image of nurse who I didn't always understand
and love deeply;

and my sisters,
Patricia, Joan, Kathleen, and *Christine;*
nurses and members of the caring profession who
taught me so much about the wear and tear of giving;
and for being who you are to me and loving me.

And in memory of my sister,
Marie,
Another nurse who loved me
and whom I miss profoundly.

This book is also dedicated in memory of my father,
Edward,
who believed in me and instilled in me that I
could do anything I set my mind to do.
Without his strength and support, my
life wouldn't be the same.

Acknowledgments

Writing this book has resulted in personal transformation and the powerful things that happened during difficult times spent hanging over my computer will always humble me. It has been a mission I could not have accomplished without the inspiration from God and the support, encouragement, and assistance of numerous people. Some of the most important people in my life stepped up to be at my side during the most challenging periods of writing.

First, thanks to my husband, Michael, for bringing great enjoyment into my life in so many ways including ballroom dancing. Your background as a ballroom dance instructor helped so much when I became stuck while using the dance metaphor for this book. You have been my dance partner for twenty years and without you, I would never have experience the love and safety I needed to be my best self.

Thanks to my son, Matthew. You filled me with great joy from the moment I experienced you. Watching you become a man has been one of the supreme pleasures of my life.

I want to thank my mother, who brought the love of nursing into my life. The days I watched you leave and come home from the hospital in your white uniform will always be fond memories.

And I thank my father for having such confidence in me. It was your love and support that helped me keep moving forward.

Thanks to my sisters, Patricia, Marie, Joan, Kathleen, and Christine, who have given me great insight about love, tension, and resistance. I am proud and happy to have had all of you in my life.

Thanks to Transformational Leadership Coaching where I received my coach training and Landmark Education where I got my life back. You taught me that it is transformation as opposed to change that frees us to experience true delight in a world that is predictably unmanageable.

I want to thank Sam Horn, who coached me through the birthing process of the idea for this book. You asked me what I was passionate about and out came the concept to combine my love of dancing and nursing into a package to help my fellow nursing colleagues. Without that lunch we spent in DC at the National Speakers Association back in November 2004, this book would not be a reality. And thanks to Dan Poynter, who provides the most wonderful books and website for writers. Your resources were extremely helpful.

I especially want to thank all my nurse friends and readers— Sharon Graham, Fran Schroeder, Frances Horton, Pamela Shaw, Susan Saunders, Pam Schroeder, Eileen Althouse, Kathy Kane, and Janette McGraw—who supported me and believed in me when I so needed it. Your perspectives and insights were invaluable contributions and I am forever grateful. I also want to thank all the nurses who took part in the nurse survey regarding their childhood background and the healthcare leaders who took part in my survey about the issues in healthcare. Your information enriched the book.

And thanks to the leaders in nursing—Jean Watson, Sandy Summers, LeAnn Thieman, Karyn Buxman, Shirley Tate Gibson, and Teresa Haller—who took the time to read and give my book their support. I value all the wonderful work you do as nursing's best. And thanks to Andrea Higham, who is a great champion for nursing through the work she does.

Thanks to Bonnie Wozniak, my coach, friend, and first editor. Without you and your support and encouragement, this book would not have gotten off the ground.

And thanks to Maureen Flanagan, who gave so generously of her time and expertise in communication. The structure of the book is definitely better because of who you are and how freely you gave of yourself.

Thanks to Christine Thorsell and Kevin Gaydosh, my publicists and friends who have made it their mission to get the word out about this book. Your encouragement to keep going when all I could see were obstacles made all the difference.

Thanks to Melanie Rigney, my editor-in-chief for taking such a personal interest in this book and me. You came into my life at the perfect time. Your wealth of knowledge and experience made *Save the First Dance for You* a much better book. Your fast friendship is appreciated.

Many thanks to Christy Jaap, my friend and proofreader who made the book a much better read. You are so generous and showed up at just the right time.

Last, but not least, thanks to George Foster for your wonderful cover design and Deb Tremper for your amazing patience and interior design.

Contents

Foreword

Jean Watson, PhD, RN, AHN-BC, FAAN
Distinguished Professor of Nursing
Murchinson-Scoville Endowed Chair in Caring Science
University of Colorado Denver and Health Sciences Center
Denver, Colorado 80262
Jean.watson@uchsc.edu

STRESS often interferes with our ability to be in transpersonal caring relationships. It can bow even the strongest and crack some under its pressure. Nurses – and those in the Caring Sciences – have the stresses of everyone else in the world plus the potential stress of serious injury to their personhood, plus to their patient, from even the slightest inaccuracy. They work with staffing shortages, requiring doing more with less. They work rotating shifts, double shifts, and return to work after 8 hours of rest to meet the needs of their patients, as well as their organizations. They're exposed to deadly diseases, accidental needlestick, and body fluid splashes.

NOW the healthcare coach, speaker, author, and self-described "Nurse Doctor" hopes to teach other nurses how to deal with stress and experience fulfillment in their work and personal lives and advise healthcare administrators about the problem. A view of nursing as a caring science helps to reframe nursing practice issues, whereby the nurse Self has to be considered as part of the professional practice plan.

"Caring science" is an emerging new field that is grounded in the discipline of nursing and evolving nursing science.

Transpersonal caring relationship moves beyond ego-self and radiates to spiritual, even cosmic concerns and connections.

Transpersonal caring calls for an authenticity of being and becoming, an ability to be present to self and other in a reflective frame; the transpersonal nurse has the ability to center consciousness and intentionality on caring, healing, and wholeness, rather than on disease, illness and pathology.

In *Save the First Dance for You—The Nurse's Guide to Serving Your Profession, Patients, and Yourself ... One Step at a Time.* Young lays out in 10 chapters several practical and coping techniques she's developed for nurses facing the challenges of today's hectic healthcare workplace and demanding home lives.

Using a dance instruction metaphor (a personal interest of the author), the book presents a 10-step program to reconcile the tensions between a nurse's calling to help and please others sometimes at the expense of their own health and happiness.

"This book is not on how to change the system, but individuals," Young says. "I wrote this book for nurses who want to redesign their day-to-day work lives, and rejuvenate the songs in their hearts and spring in their steps.

Young's central premise is that nurses often put other people's needs first and their own needs last, and that can cause the nurse to wear out physically and emotionally. Within a view of advancing nurse's Self, nurses can further advance caring –healing practices for others.

Chapters in the book cover such topics as: preventing burnout by engaging in self-caring practices first; learning to adhere to values and principles, yet flexible when dealing with ambiguity, dynamics of humanity and individuals as well as paradoxical situations; viewing all situations as opportunities for growth; setting goals and taking action; knowing the roles of being a leader and a follower; learning about yourself through caring-healing relationships; how beliefs act as filters that create our experiences; freeing oneself to have fun; being authentic; and "strutting your stuff."

While primarily written for the nursing profession, other healthcare workers and even employees in other industries can benefit from Young's 10-step approach to work-home balance.

Doris L. Young, Ph. D., known as "The Nurse Doctor," has been a nurse for 30 years and has served in surgical and trauma units and behavioral units at major hospitals. As a nurse and nursing leader, Dr. Young has faced these issues personally. Dr. Young has taught people within healthcare and other industries how to deal with stress and experience fulfillment in their work and personal life.

If you are frustrated with all the trying nursing encounters you are required to deal with daily, you need this book. If you follow these guidelines, you will achieve the foundational consciousness required for wholeness and transpersonal caring.

Introduction

As a girl, I asked my mother for dance lessons. She reasoned that if I received them, my five sisters would have to have them as well. So, I settled for watching my girlfriends take dance lessons every Saturday. I sat loyally along the wall each weekend and danced in my mind and soul, but never with my feet.

I loved their costumes and the music. Some had pink leotards with pink tutus and pink slippers. Others had black leotards and black tap shoes. I could see myself dancing with them. I could feel the music inside me. But I never stepped onto that dance floor.

One day, while studying for exams at my girlfriend's house, her mother encouraged me to dress up in my friend's leotard, tutu and dance slippers. I jumped at the idea. I was in heaven as I bounded around the room.

Seeing my joy, the mother suggested I wear it home to show my parents. Since I was supposed to be studying and not playing, I was afraid this might upset them. But I couldn't resist.

I walked home like a princess in the most wonderful costume in the world. But my parents felt otherwise, and I was never allowed to study with my friend again.

I didn't pursue dance as a grown-up because I felt there was no use in trying to fill an empty part of my childhood that I had locked away and given up on.

I was wrong.

Finally, I signed up for a ballet exercise class. I was surprised when the instructor told me I had the perfect feet for ballet. I wondered what might have happened had I taken those dance lessons as a girl.

My class rejuvenated me and flooded me with a new sense of joy—like when the Grinch's heart grew ten times its size.

Sadly, this didn't last very long, because my instructor got sick and stopped giving lessons.

Once again, I had to put my dream of dancing on hold.

Then a man who would eventually become my husband asked me to dance. He introduced himself as a professional ballroom dance instructor. I thought I'd died and gone to heaven. How was I so lucky?

Over the years, we've danced away the emptiness created by my childhood.

When I dance, I'm floating above the world. The music becomes part of me, my feet glide along the floor, and my body moves smoothly in perfect balance with my husband. We move in perfect symmetry and become one with the music—two birds in flight, with music guiding our movements.

The good thing about passion is that it can be found in more than one area. As a girl, I also dreamed of being a nurse. I can remember looking in the mirror and saying to myself, "I'm going to be a nurse."

Seeing myself in my nursing uniform for the first time, I was sure I had fulfilled my destiny. All was well inside and out.

I loved watching nurses do what they loved. It's just like watching someone on the dance floor who's in beautiful harmony with the music. Seeing someone obviously having fun is uplifting; watching a nurse expressing her love and compassion is inspiring.

I want to help you keep your feeling of passion for your profession. When dancers aren't in sync, or a nurse is just going through the motions, it's painful—painful to see, and even more painful to experience.

Nursing is a serving profession. As a person who serves others, you often put everyone else's needs first and your own last.

If you stay on this path, it will wear you out and our profession will lose your matchless gifts.

This book is written to help you, as a nurse, redesign your day-to-day work life to rejuvenate the sound of music in your heart. Using the dancing metaphor, this book is a ten-step program on how to get your own rhythm back.

It's your opportunity to remember why you came into the nursing profession in the first place. It wasn't a decision you made lightly. People who go into nursing want to help others. They love nurturing and caring for others. They're patient and kind, until their strength is overused and becomes their weakness.

This is *not* a book on how to change systemically, but individually. We can't change the whole system at once, but what we can do is change ourselves. Each of us has control over only one thing—our response to what happens to us. As we transform individually, we can transform our homes, our work team, our organization, and the entire healthcare system.

My sincere hope is that this book will be like a lifeline for you—an emotional intravenous feeding, if you will. Once, I became dehydrated after a viral illness and was given intravenous fluids. I can remember feeling the life come back into my body as the needed fluids were provided. The nursing profession can be emotionally dehydrating, and my goal is to replenish the fluid it depletes.

I.

Save the First Dance for You

Dance is the hidden language of the soul.
Martha Graham (1893-1991)

At a ballroom dance exhibition, I watched a graceful couple move around the dance floor. They moved apart, came together, and performed the same steps in perfect synchronization to the music and to each other. As one glided backward, the other moved forward. They turned; they dipped, and moved in unison. In my mind's eye, I saw myself floating around the floor and I was sure it wouldn't take long before I looked just like them. Of course, a six-week group class does not a beautiful dancer make. Only the truly accomplished can move through the steps with ease.

That's true in life as well as on the dance floor. Whether or not we are aware of it, we are always dancing. All the people in our relationships at home, with friends, or on the job are dance partners. We could either flow with them, enjoy the dance, or we thwart the current and the dance becomes a power struggle of pushing, pulling and resistance.

How would your life be if you where able to take
care of yourself, had more energy, and felt fulfilled
by your personal and professional life?

As nurses we know how to take care of everyone, often at our own expense. Our plates are full of so many wonderful things to do and accomplish. It's easy to put ourselves on the back burner. However, it's vital to acknowledge you have a right, in fact a need, to honor and nurture yourself while you take care of others. In turn, when you give yourself permission to take care of yourself, you give the same permission to everyone else. I encourage you to move past your guilt or unease and accept that you're worthy and deserve to be self-fulfilled. It's important for you to believe you can have what you want. Then, give yourself the freedom to ask for and fulfill the desires of your heart.

One nurse began to feel tired of listening to her colleagues' complaining in the lounge about each other, the nurse manager, and their husbands. She wanted to play a new role on the unit, so she decided to stop being part of the gossip. When a staff member came to complain about someone else, she took the opportunity to ask if the complainer had spoken with the person. She also offered to role-play their conversation. Not long after she started doing this, she began to notice people stopped coming to talk with her. Soon other staff members began to stop gossiping. It didn't take long before no one was complaining without making a plan to work out the issue. Eventually, the staff became more solution-focused, supportive, and it wasn't long before the group started having more social gatherings and interacting like an innovative team.

Another nurse felt exhausted and started noticing she was making errors at work. She identified her compulsion to take care of others, which gave her no time for herself. Everything felt like a duty, even getting together with friends. She felt resentment toward her husband and kids. She wanted to do arts and crafts and enjoy reading on her days off, but felt guilty whenever she took time for herself. At our first coaching session, she decided to take a half-day on her next day off and enjoy arts and crafts.

She found she was so energized the next day that she also actually enjoyed doing her chores. She knew she was on to something. She also had told herself she had no time for exercise, though she knew it would catch up with her one day. As she explored this further, she discovered her mother had taught her it was selfish to take care of herself. She began to distinguish her unjustified guilt. Her hardest struggle was to do self-fulfilling things in spite of her feelings of guilt. She kept a journal of her experiences. When she finally overcame her guilt, she took mornings off from her chores on her day off at least once a week and did arts and crafts while she did her laundry. She was amazed at how much more energy she had and how much less resentment she felt. She became more rested and the mistakes stopped.

I have experienced the wonderful movements of the nursing dance for thirty years. My call began at ten. I have had my graceful moments as well as times when I have been out of sync. These experiences have taught me what it means to be a nurse. I love nursing deeply with the fullness and respect that only comes from seasoning and maturity. It is now my great privilege to be a coach for nurses and share the steps to have less stress, more energy, and more fulfillments in their personal and professional life.

Nursing Dance: Master the First Steps

Wisdom began to form on the night of my first experience in the emergency room. I was in my second year of nursing school. A woman rushed toward me with a big bundle in her arms, screaming, "Help me! Help me! My baby has a fever. She was shaking, and now she won't answer me."

I quickly guided them to a nearby stretcher and called for the doctor. After his examination, he determined that the baby had had a seizure. He ordered 0.2 cc of Phenobarbital and a Tylenol suppository. The LPN on that night brought in the medication and gave it to the little girl. I stayed with her with my hand on her belly, rocking her. Suddenly, I realized I couldn't feel her breathing. I yelled, "She's not breathing. We need help!"

As the staff came rushing in with the crash cart, they performed as a precision team. Each one danced their part, and the baby had IVs and life back in her body within moments.

I stood paralyzed, watching the miracle of modern medicine. The baby's first breath on her own seemed like the first breath I had taken since it all started. She became stable, and we admitted her to the pediatric unit.

At our nightly post-conference, the instructor told us that the incident happened because the baby had been given 2 cc of Phenobarbital instead of 0.2 cc. She had gone into respiratory arrest because a nurse had made a mistake.

My heart stopped for a moment. That night, I made an absolute commitment to myself and to all the people I would ever care for that nothing would happen to another human being that I could prevent. I became hyper vigilant.

I soon found out that it takes a long time to gain the expertise to make that vow possible. It takes years of school and practice before a nurse can feel totally competent. What does that mean? Let me count the ways.

A nurse must be proficient at a variety of medical treatments, have a firm understanding of an array of healthcare functions and a background in individual and family psychology.

A nurse must have an awareness of the complex interactions throughout the departments in a hospital or healthcare organization.

A nurse has to keep meticulous records, even in emergency situations, and communicate precise information to numerous administrative areas and people.

A nurse has to know how to evade the bureaucracy when test results are processed too slowly and how to initiate reevaluation of care when something is amiss.

Given the emphasis on cost containment, a nurse must focus on monetary expenditures and, need I say, computer skills in our wish to be "paperless."

As the foundation of all these skills, however, a nurse requires self-assurance and the character to maintain equilibrium when faced with the various demands of physicians, other hospital staff, patients, and families. Confidence is a must.

Execution of so many diverse skills, coupled with the need for a great attitude places great demands on the individual nurse. Sometimes, the demands are just too great.

Nursing Dance: Massage Your Sore Feet

Nursing is not just a job. It's a calling and a way of being that offers the satisfaction of serving others with consideration and kindness. However, let's face it—nursing is still a job. There are some days when it is just plain hard. Those are the kinds of days when the only reason to show up is to get a paycheck. Now, it is not unreasonable to expect a paycheck for services rendered. However, if the paycheck becomes the *only* reason for going to work, burnout is on the horizon.

I found myself in a state of exhaustion after twenty-five years of nursing. I was working as the director of surgical services, and I felt that if one more person asked me for something, I was going to tell him or her where to take that request. This was very different than my normal attitude that the "buck stops here." I was tired and resentful. I had to drag myself to work and give myself an attitude adjustment just before I walked in the door. I now know that the name for this state is burnout.

Burnout usually occurs after people have given all they can and the well is empty the next time they go searching for the energy to take an extra shift or put up with an inconsiderate colleague. "What about me?" is a perfectly reasonable response when the job seems to be all about others with little recognition of your own needs or contributions.

The toll can be great. Being hyper vigilant is exhausting and can result in giving from your fabric, from your essence rather than your excess. This is draining. If you don't save the first dance for you, you're going to wind up leaving the profession and that is a tragedy.

How do you avoid burnout—or move beyond it?

Because nursing is demanding, it is important to know what gives you energy and what drains your energy. It is important to recharge on a regular basis or you will be discharged. My drive to write this book was fueled by the realization that we must take care of ourselves if we are going to be able to take care of the people we serve. I also realized that we are sabotaging our own happiness.

In her book *Approval Addiction,* Joyce Meyer talks about people-pleasers who feel wonderful when comforting and pleasing those in need. They unconsciously crave the emotional rewards of service, and this becomes the focus of their lives.

Unfortunately, nurses are prime candidates to become compulsive people-pleasers. Nursing requires giving and nurturing. If you didn't have these qualities, you would not be a good candidate for the job. Nurses take care of people in need and so you are compelled to do things right. Because innocent lives depend on you, you are a relentless watchdog whether on duty or off.

You are more than willing to set aside your own authentic needs and over give, not realizing that denying them can have severe consequences.

Sound familiar? If so, then you're probably eager to know how this damaging behavior starts.

People-pleasers are often raised in families where needs and feelings are not valued, respected, or important. As children, people-pleasers are expected to take care of others' needs and are recognized for doing so. The affirmation feels so good that the behavior continues until it becomes the only way to get attention and advancement.

This means that below your level of consciousness, you really want people to be happy with you because that is the only way you are happy with yourself. This perspective is the drive of the people-pleaser. It is very subtle, so don't be fooled.

How it starts, however, is not nearly as important as how it stops. As a nurse, you must stay in touch with your driving force and innermost desires to counter your compulsive people-pleasing tendencies.

Ask yourself: What do you want in return for what you give?

I can remember the first time someone asked me *what I wanted*. It was as if someone had just turned on a light bulb. I had no idea what I wanted. It never even occurred to me to have "wants." I was so aware of what everyone else needed that I was completely unaware of myself. I didn't expect, nor was I capable of knowing or receiving, what I wanted. It took me years to unwind from this mind-set.

What do *you* want?

You bring a magnificent gift to the world as a nurse and you can only keep giving if your cup has something in it. To keep your cup full, you must revitalize and enjoy yourself. Receiving while you're giving is a natural process and yet, for many of us, it requires development. You don't have to be demanding toward someone else to be giving to yourself. All you need is time and space for yourself. All it takes is honoring yourself enough to take it. Be totally sincere in your effort to answer the question of what's in it for you. Your physical, emotional, and spiritual health depends on it. We all need acknowledgement, appreciation, and pleasure. Denying these needs leads to volatile results and exhaustion.

As we explore where you are on the path to living the life you dream of, I want you to feel the pure joy of our time together. I know how special you are and how important you are to this time and place. Your well-being not only affects you and your friends, family, and the people with whom you come in direct contact; it also influences every person who comes in contact with those people, and the people those people touch, and so on. You have a huge impact on the world just doing your everyday activities, so take care of yourself.

Nursing Dance: **Three Cs**

Let's start our journey by exploring the three Cs. When I am speaking to an audience of nurses, I ask them three questions so I can get to know them better. I would like to ask you those questions, but first I want you to know it's a fixed quiz. I want you to answer yes to all three questions. As you say YES, put your right arm up in the air and seize a great big piece of the universe and pull it to you. Here goes!

Would you like to have less stress in your life?

Would you like to have more energy?

Finally and most importantly,

Are you willing to make the commitment to the necessary alterations to have less stress and more energy?

If you answered YES to all three questions, you have just demonstrated the first characteristic of the most stress-hardy people as identified by Joan Borysenko of Harvard University. People who make a commitment—the first C—can sustain more stress and are more successful. When I think of commitment, I think of a woman named Helen I worked with while I was director of surgical services. Helen put our instrument tray together. One day, she said, "When I put an instrument tray together, I am saving a life. Somebody's mamma may need that instrument tray, and I am saving somebody's mamma."

Helen inspired me. She really knew about commitment. She took what could have been a boring job and saw its importance. She didn't see a string of instruments; she saw people's lives in her hands. If we could all see how we fit into the bigger picture and stayed interested, wouldn't life feel better? Wouldn't we be able to make a bigger contribution? Wouldn't we be able to sustain any hardship if we knew the importance of what we do?

Control is the second C. In one year, my sister, Kathy, lost her husband and found out she had a life-threatening illness. Not knowing what she would hear on the day she received her diagnosis, she planned to go to an amusement park. She determined her only other choice was to stay home alone, so she went to the park.

It was on the roller coaster as she clicked up to the first drop-off that she reasoned, "Isn't life like a roller coaster? It has ups and downs, twists and turns, and you never know exactly what is going to happen next. Ultimately, we know the ride will come to a stop. I like roller coasters and I am going to live my life even though I don't know what is in store. I will love my children and enjoy every moment I have."

She has been such a blessing to so many. And when she felt confident she would survive, she went to nursing school. Her children have grown and graduated from high school and married. Kathy is now the fifth nurse in our family today.

The final C is challenge. If we can look at obstacles as challenges to get over, around, or through, we will be more stress-hardy and successful. This really hit home for me one Labor Day weekend. We had had a hurricane the week before and the surf was a little rougher then usual. My husband and my girlfriend's husband were out in the water while my friend and I were doing our usual sunbathing.

I had this intense desire to go in the water and I couldn't convince my girlfriend to go with me. I was determined to overcome my fear intensified by seeing the movie *Jaws* so many years ago. I got in as far as the breakers and froze.

You know what happened next. I got knocked over by a huge wave. After the washing machine wave spit me out toward the shore, I got up, pulled the hair out of my face, and waved at my friend as if I meant to do that. Then I looked up and on a deck of a nearby home I saw a man with a pair of binoculars looking directly at me. I looked down and realized my bathing attire was not longer in its proper position, if you know what I mean.

It was that moment that I realized there are predators on land as well as in the sea and I wasn't going to let them stop me from doing what I wanted to do. I got through the breakers, reached my husband, and had the best time I'd had in years. I felt as if I were ten years old again. It was a great day, and I have never been sorry about choosing to accept fear as a challenge to overcome. It makes us strong and resilient each time we recognize our fear and do what we want anyway.

As you begin to look at your dreams as real possibilities, recognize that with commitment anything is achievable. Embrace the awareness of controlling the way you live your life in spite of ever-present adversity. Allow the challenges you face to make you robust and to see fear as a reality of life, not as an obstacle to your accomplishments. With all this ahead, you need energy, so it is extremely important to learn to relax.

Nursing Dance: **Learn to Relax**

(1) Start waking up just fifteen minutes early. In a quiet space, direct your breathing to the different parts of your body, starting at your feet. Once you have relaxed your body, take yourself to your personal place of relaxation. Go to the mountains or the beach. Imagine being in this peaceful place and notice what is going on around you. Become aware of what you hear and then observe what you see in your personal space of relaxation. When you are fully relaxed, begin to imagine yourself having your dream reality. Experience the joy of knowing you can have what you want.

Doing this every morning and again in the evening releases the muscles from habitual, unconscious tension. Mentally observing and letting go of troubling, worrisome thoughts are necessary for relaxation. We must learn to "let go" on a deeper level than we are accustomed to. Adding the awareness of creating new possibilities will make room for them.

(2) When you feel tired from a long day, it may not take much to rebalance. Notice what you are saying to yourself. This sound is the music you are dancing to. Are you listing all the things you have to do, or are you recognizing the blessings in your life? If everything that comes to mind is a task, write the list on paper. Put a plus sign next to things that energize you and a minus sign next to the things that drain you. Make a column next to this list and put down what you can do to balance the minuses. For every item on your list that drains you, put down something that energizes you. Stay with this process until you feel a peacefulness come over you, the sense that all is well inside and out.

Nursing Dance: Be Honest with Others

(1) It's hard to relax when the to-do list keeps getting longer and longer. If you take on more than you realistically can handle, you'll wind up resenting the added responsibilities. However, the prospect of saying "No" to those who ask for or need help is awful too. What to do? Honesty is the only way out of the cycle of resentment and fear.

It feels great when we are honestly saying "Yes" when we want to do something and saying "No" when we don't. Take time to find a peaceful feeling about what you are about to do. If you don't feel at peace with something, take a moment and express yourself.

Personal honesty is the first step toward acceptance. Everything you build in your life is according to your own specifications. If you choose not to give people what they want and they become unhappy, it is not your responsibility.

Being open with your desires, feelings, and thoughts will lead you to the truth of what you want. A healthy relationship requires candor, even if other people don't want to hear the truth because it doesn't get them what they want.

(2) Beware of developing a false sense of accountability. You have enough liability for yourself without taking on blame for others. People-pleasers will push themselves if they think it means everyone will be happy with them. Too often, people take advantage of us if we let them. Part of the human disposition is to do so. Don't rely on others to treat you justly and sincerely.

(3) If someone asks for something, you get to decide whether you want to do it. Just because it is hard for you to say no doesn't mean that they shouldn't ask. Being a people-pleaser means you are not focusing on you correctly. Having difficulty saying no makes you susceptible. Thinking you should do what people ask puts you at risk. Shifting a "no" to a "yes" if someone gets angry makes things worse.

Begin making the shift by seeing it as a great opportunity to take care of you when someone asks for something. Learn to say "Thank you for thinking of me, but my plate is full right now." Or respond, "I feel honored that you asked, but I just can't fit this in right now." If it's your family, explain, "I can't fit that into my schedule today. Is there another way you can accomplish that?"

(4) *Spend time with your emotions and begin to contemplate how you are creating your experience. Maybe you will find that you haven't clearly asked for what you want because you're not aware of precisely what you want. Recognizing your emotional response will help get you in touch with what you want. Embrace your feelings rather than dismissing them as negative. Resist blaming other people for your emotions. Feel them and honor them. Examine what they are telling you about yourself.*

Perhaps you'll become aware that you give in after asking for what you want so that the other person never has to respond. You may be frightened or think it's futile to ask for what you want.

Maybe you only know how to give, not how to receive. Maybe you really don't value yourself enough, so you question your desire. You can be so focused outside yourself that you don't realize that you even have wants.

Nursing Dance: Be Honest with Yourself

Honesty doesn't simply apply to being honest with others. It has to begin within us. It is indispensable to be open to the possibility of developing a wonderful dance with ourselves. We cannot comfortably dance with anyone else until we know our own dance. To know our own dance is to begin the process of healing our soul and embracing our true essence. We see the outside dance world through our own dance. We have a certain dance pattern that persists no matter who we dance with. We don't really know the people in our lives. We only know the way they look through our dance patterns.

During our nursing dance with others, it is comfortable and easy to see what needs to be fixed in them. However, our relationships with our dance partners are the most valuable way to learn about who we truly are. Here is how the dance goes. If we notice a problem in someone close to us and don't see it in ourselves, it is a part of our dance that we have disowned or denied. Psychologists call this projection. You know you have a limp in your dance step if you get upset at others for their limitations. As dancers in life, we continue to view the people around us as mirrors of our rejected self until we heal the split in ourselves. Healing is merely the process of complete acceptance. The way out of this house of mirrors is to be willing to admit that we have the characteristic we find unacceptable or wonderful in others. Next, we must be open to possibility of embracing and creating something new with those characteristics that are inconsistent with our concept of ourselves.

One exercise I found in "*Receiving Love*" by Harville Hendrix and Helen Lakelly Hunt may be very helpful in recovering the "unknown" part of us.

Make a list of all the characteristics you see in people closest to you. You may also ask other people to give you characteristics they see in you. Note whether you see the characteristic as positive or negative and list them separately. Then look for the positive characteristic within yourself. These are the traits that you may have disowned. Take time to embrace them.

Next, take the negative characteristics and create a positive affirmation you want to own. For example, if you see your negative characteristic as defensiveness, you would write the affirmation, "I am open-minded" or "I am accepting."

This process may not be without effort, but it does bear great fruit. You will feel a great freeing of your spirit when you do. When you freely accept yourself, you are able to accept others as well. In the spirit of acceptance, you will be able to ask for what you want and accept that your dance partner has a choice in whether to comply with your request.

Nursing Dance: Take Ownership

As nurses, how often are we asked to do things we don't really want to do? It might be covering a shift; skipping lunch; or ignoring a physician, manager, or colleague's unkind words or lack of assistance. We go along, say nothing, and focus on getting the job done, being nice, and avoiding conflict.

You've all heard that people can't take advantage of you unless you allow it to happen. For years I wondered how it can be our responsibility when other people are uncaring, disrespectful, or unkind.

Then I learned that we can only own what we think, say, and do. It is possible to tell people you don't like something they've done without feeling angry. In the past, I frequently said nothing until anger gave me the energy to voice my opinion. The eruption coming from anger would usually be greeted with a negative response.

Our choice of response has consequences. If someone asks us to do something, we have every right to say yes or no. The other person may or may not be happy about the choice. It is our choices as well as our view and our dance that we own. Every time we experience another person, we have an opportunity to identify our limits and become aware of how we see the world. If we hope our dance partner will point out when our life is out of balance and accommodate us, our expectations will probably go unmet. When we take responsibility for allowing the necessary transformation within ourselves, we create a space for something new.

The first step is to separate ourselves physically or emotionally from any person with whom we're struggling. When we have some space, we can analyze our part in the situation. When we identify what we want, we can ask for it. If our request is ignored, we can make the separation permanent or decide our next action. Making these choices takes some time while we consider all the elements of the situation. We may have to look at how we ask. Do we need anger to get the guts up to ask? If so, it probably comes out as a demand. As we heal, we can ask for more and demand less.

We must ask ourselves if we've asked in a non-demanding way. After our healing, we determine if we're getting what we want and if our relationship is worth saving. If we make this decision quickly, we will be sorry because things often seem impossible and our belief causes us to give up. We create possibilities through our beliefs. Once we take full responsibility for our actions and feelings we may see things much more clearly.

Nursing Dance: **Learn How to Open Up**

The Johari Window, named for its inventors, Joseph Luft and Harry Ingham, is a wonderful illustration of the human interaction process. The model uses a four-paned "window" that divides personal awareness into open, hidden, blind, and unknown quadrants. The lines dividing the four panes are like window shades that can move as an interaction progresses.

Johari Window	Known to Self	Not Known to Self
Known to Others	Open	Blind
Not Known to Others	Hidden	Unknown

The open quadrant represents things that both others know and we know about ourselves. For example, if we meet on the street, I know the color of your hair and so do you. This window represents feelings, motives, behaviors, wants, needs, desires, or any other factual information that describe who you are. When we meet someone new, the open quadrant is small. As the process of getting to know one another continues, we exchange information and the quadrant grows.

The blind quadrant represents things others know about us that are not known to us. Let's say you come to a meeting with lint on the back of your suit. This information is in your blind quadrant because others see it, but not you. If someone tells you, then this information becomes a part of your open quadrant. Blind spots can be found in other, more involved areas.

For example, if we're having a conversation, someone may notice that I am not making eye contact. The person may not say anything, not wanting to embarrass me, but draws his or her own conclusion that I am being insincere. How can I discover more about our relationship and myself? I may notice a slight hesitation, and possibly ask a question. If I don't notice, or don't get a direct answer when I ask, I will never become aware of what is going on between us.

The hidden quadrant contains information that we know about ourselves that others do not know. If we do not tell anyone our favorite dessert, this information is in our hidden quadrant. If I tell someone that I love Crème Brule, my hidden quadrant reduces and my open quadrant expands. In effect, I have my whole life's story to share with others as we get to know and trust each other. The hidden quadrant expands through the process of self-disclosure.

The final quadrant is called unknown because it represents things that neither we nor others know about us. If I describe a dream that I had, we may both attempt to understand its significance. A new awareness may emerge, known to neither of us before our conversation. Our unknown quadrant reduces while our open quadrant increases. New situations offer opportunities to reveal additional information.

Recently, I learned that I have a form of dyslexia that only occurs under stress. This information decreased my unknown quadrant and expanded my open quadrant with the person who identified it. It has been in my hidden quadrant until I decided to share it here and now it is in my open quadrant with all of you. Knowing this information clarified why I had so much difficulty reading for timed-reading tests or in front of the class as a child.

Thus, new situations can trigger a new awareness and personal growth. When we expand our unknown quadrant, we are changing our filters, breaking old patterns, and releasing ourselves of self-imposed bondage.

The process of moving previously unknown information into the open quadrant has been equated to Maslow's concept of self-actualization. Once people reach a level of self-actualization, they tend to have more peak experiences than the average person. A peak experience is one that takes you out of yourself and makes you feel one with life or nature or God. These experiences are known to transform people, and many people actively seek them out for guidance.

Maslow identified qualities that seemed to be associated with self-actualization. People in this group have a strong desire for truth, goodness, beauty, unity, wholeness, and transcendence. They thrive with a sense of aliveness, uniqueness, completion, justice, and order. And they experience a deep enjoyment of simplicity, environmental richness, effortlessness, playfulness, self-sufficiency, and meaningfulness.

As nurses, we desire these experiences for the world as well as ourselves. Our goal is to have them on a regular basis, and that requires making time and space. Unfortunately, there are many people who live in poverty and worry about getting enough to eat and a safe place to live. In fact, Maslow supposed that many of the issues in the world today stemmed from the fact that people haven't had their basic needs met.

Increasing the size of our open quadrant is a win-win proposition. Becoming more self-aware creates the opportunity to become more self-accepting. Self-acceptance leads to more openness and sharing. The more we share with trusted friends or our spouse, the more these people can help us expand our self-knowledge. The more we know about ourselves and accept ourselves, the better our relationships can be.

Nursing Dance: **Allow Time for Healing**

As nurses, we spend so much time helping others heal their emotional and physical wounds that there is little time for our own healing. Yet we all need to heal. As we experience healing of our old emotional wounds, we give other people permission to heal theirs. We can start by becoming aware of our strengths and weaknesses. As we get more in touch with our inner wisdom, we become more open to others and less judgmental.

We all judge the world and people's behavior according to our own interpretation of what is right. Identifying the motivation you and others have leads to better understanding. With increased reflection, we become more respectful of differences. This perspective produces the seeds for success.

As we learn to appreciate our differences, we begin to be grateful for what others bring. When we are thankful for and value the gift each person brings, we can benefit from the wealth of wisdom and expertise they have to share and enjoy a smoother experience. Even if we are in uncharted waters, we can accomplish great things.

Nursing Dance: **Know the Stages of Healing**

As you read this book, I know that you will experience many feelings. Some of you are reading to prevent burnout while others are trying to move from burnout to healing. Elisabeth Kübler-

Ross identified the stages underlying all transformation, and it's important to be prepared for them.

(a) The first stage is denial, which is a temporary defense that gives time to prepare for acceptance of what will come later. Long-term denial can be very costly.

(b) Anger is the phase that occurs when you realize some things have to go.

(c) The third stage is bargaining, mostly with God, to take away the difficulty.

(d) Next is sadness/despair, when energy becomes low and hope is almost lost.

(e) The fifth stage is acceptance, when you see yourself most clearly and make the necessary choices to facilitate transformation and healing.

(f) You will eventually reach a time of rebirth and delight as you replace old experiences with new thinking.

(g) The last stage is creating a new life. Creating new possibilities for you and your life on the inside automatically leads to external transformation.

How do you take care of yourself? My wish for each of you is to take time for self-care because you deserve it and, even more importantly, you need it. Your ability to help others is only as good as your ability to keep yourself strong and healthy. We need you in our profession. Your patients need you. Your family needs you. And you need you.

The full magnitude of being aware and accepting can be seen through increased flexibility and agility. A ballroom dancer who becomes conscious of all the elements in fine dancing sashays through varied routines. A nurse can soar through intricate circumstances by becoming conscious of the basic essence of who he or she really is. When you save the first dance for you, you allow yourself to establish your frame of reference, which is foundational. Learning to bend your knees and establish your frame will help you dance with ease. We will find out how in the next chapter.

Questions to Explore

1. What is your passion in life? Or, what makes you happiest and most fulfilled?

2. What do you want? List at least five things.

3. What do you need? List at least five things.

4. What are your favorite pastimes? List at least five things.

5. What would you like to do or accomplish (personally or professionally) to consider your life to have been well-lived?

To receive your free gift worth $29 go to
http://www.SavetheFirstDanceforYou.com/relaxation.htm

II.

Bend Your Knees/
Establish Your Dance Frame

*The dancer's body is simply the
luminous manifestation of the soul.*
Isadora Duncan (1878-1927)

I was standing in an enormous room surrounded by wall-to-wall mirrors from ceiling to floor and my dance instructor said, "Let's begin with a demonstration of dance frame." He pointed down at his bent knees and said, "Bend your knees." He explained that this flex would keep my upper body steady by absorbing all the shock from the movement of a dance.

"Now, hold your abdomen in as you raise your chest and relax your shoulders. Imagine a string extending from your head while you keep everything loose and flexible."

Holding in my belly had a profound effect on my chest. Letting go of my shoulders required a little more practice. The string effect took a little longer, but once I got the hang of it, I actually felt like I was floating.

Next, he brought my arms up to right angles at my shoulders. He explained that after I learned the steps, a partner would fill in the space my arms created. He told me I would learn to maintain the position while I moved through the dance steps and held resistance against my partner.

All this and I hadn't learned my first step! Before taking one stride, I had to master the foundational principles of dance. I was captivated.

The beginning of my first dance lesson taught me not only how I need to prepare for dance, but also how much this is true about anything in life.

Groundwork is so important.

> *How would your life be*
> *if you were firm on the inside about your values*
> *and principles and flexible on the outside*
> *about how you dealt with people and situations?*

Nurses often want to help everyone feel good, even if it's at their own expense. We must get to know our limits or we will be pushed past our boundaries. Become aware of what you value and aspire to. This starts by focusing inward and moving past our internal struggles to influence the outside world.

One nurse was slapped on the butt by a doctor. She discussed the situation with other nurses, but never said anything to the doctor. Instead, she tried to have her schedule changed so she would never have to work with him again. During coaching, she clarified her value of mutual respect in relationships. By accepting this physician's behavior without response, she allowed him to be disrespectful. She realized she didn't respect herself and therefore allowed the doctor to push past her boundaries. It became clear what she wanted to do. She informed her nurse manager and described her expectations to the physician the next time she saw him. She also went to the joint practice committee of the hospital and reported the incident just in case it was happening to anyone else. As the story unfolded, she shared her history of sexual abuse and felt she was standing up for herself for the first time in her life. As she healed her residual feelings from her sexual abuse as a child, she became an advocate for nurses honoring themselves.

In another situation, a new operating room nurse noticed that she and another more senior nurse were scheduled for more weekends than the other nurses. Initially, she thought it was just a coincidence, but it continued. She talked with the other nurse, who shared that it had been happening to her for a long time, but that she had always feared retribution if she complained. She greatly valued her free time on the weekends with her family, yet worried that her colleague might be right. After some soul-searching and verification of schedules, she decided to ask her manager about the situation without making any assumptions. To her astonishment, her manager had never looked at the number of weekends each person worked because she used a rotation template to create the schedule. Both she and her colleague were pleasantly surprised at how easy it was to change their schedules.

So many things are unconsciously established in childhood without a foundation. In dance, you must develop a strong emotional foundation with your balanced frame to maintain equilibrium while moving across the floor with your dance partner. In nursing, you must also build a strong emotional foundation and a balanced frame of reference to maintain equilibrium while moving through your daily tasks with your care partner.

Nursing Dance: Establish Your Foundation

Imagine nursing as a dance in which you need to be aware of your structure before beginning. Great steadiness and flexibility are derived from knowing yourself well and having awareness about your motivation and intention. You need to know where you stand, what you value, where you want to go, and how you want to get there.

If this sounds self-centered to you, then know that it is possible to be firm on the inside about your convictions and flexible on the outside when interacting with others. Control lies within your inner sense of knowing. In both dance and nursing, this steadiness and flexibility take time to achieve.

Nursing Dance: Self-awareness

Becoming self-aware is a complex process that involves minute attention to the fact that all of us need to be our own reference point. We must learn to recognize what is called our *soul position*. If another person sets the pace, the pace is always subject to change without our input or consideration. It is based on someone else's needs and desires, devoid of our personal stamp.

How do you go about perceiving who you really are on the inside? When determining what you want for yourself or when being asked to fulfill the needs of others, ask yourself two questions: *What am I willing to do and give? What am I not willing to do or give?* When you are fulfilled, you know your source of control and have much more to give to others.

Even if you've been a nurse for many years, you may not know what it takes to maintain a healthy frame because we are not taught to take care of ourselves. We are taught to take care of others, even at our own expense. We may think that we will receive what we give, but this process is not automatic.

Nursing Dance: Know Your Intention

Becoming emotionally aware requires that we understand our intentions.

All of us have specific intentions about what we want to achieve. These may be conscious or unconscious. Most nurses and people in the helping professions think that they chose their profession because they want to help others. Of course! We spend time thinking about and often intuitively knowing what others need. We often provide things without being asked. We generally enjoy doing for others.

Over time, however, we begin to want something back. We may be hurt if people don't reciprocate or appreciate what we do for them.

People may even lash out at us for giving help they haven't requested. This leads us to think that these ungrateful people are hurtful and insensitive.

The result is a cycle of action and resentment and a sequence of hurt. We are either being hurt, being afraid of being hurt, being angry about being hurt, or withdrawing from others because of being hurt.

The only way out of this circular wounding is to understand the role you play. Becoming conscious of your motivation for helping others is critical. Perhaps helping people was a source of affirmation as a child and continues to make you feel good about your contribution to the world. It's equally possible, however, that it may not be only about the enjoyment of helping people.

Nursing Dance: **Dealing with Fear**

Let's look beneath the surface. We grow up learning to fear all kind of things. We fear failure, rejection, loneliness, embarrassment, judgment, and even success.

We develop anxiety in response to all kinds of fears. We learn this emotional reaction from our parents, teachers, or the bully down the street. If they tell us in words or actions that we are not OK, we develop a fear of repeating that feeling of rejection.

Fears cause a repetitive response to situations with behavior patterns that really don't serve us. Our fear of rejection can result in a compulsive drive to please everyone in our life.

This leads to overdoing and being more helpful than we really want to be. Too often, we have no idea this is happening. We can't seem to stop, even if we become aware of the problem, because it's a habit that may have started as a way of staying safe in our early childhood. The end result is that our self-worth and self-love are based on whether we feel loved by the people important to us.

I remember trying to stop volunteering for things I didn't want to do. I would see myself offering to do things just because at the moment it sounded like a good idea. I felt stupid because a "yes" would come out of my mouth and I would then feel obligated to follow through. If helping others is the only way we know to please others, it becomes a compulsion.

Nursing Dance: **It's Not About You**

Everyone has experienced a time in his or her life of feeling unloved or unaccepted. When we don't feel loved, we will eventually feel unlovable. People deal with this differently. Some people shy away from others to protect themselves; others become outgoing and try to win others over. Nurses are usually the latter.

People often believe that they weren't accepted because they did something wrong or something is wrong with them. The reality is that people will respond to us based on their frame of reference, which has very little to do with us.

When we come to the realization that what other people think doesn't make it so, we can free ourselves from the overwhelming need to make everyone happy.

The good news is that this fear doesn't have to continue to control our lives. We can decide to discontinue a certain behavior and make a commitment to a new way of being. We have the freedom and the power to choose.

We may choose to stay away from a person or ask for different behavior. We have a choice about the meaning we place on the situation. We have a choice about our response as well as a choice about the people with whom we associate. Choosing takes courage, particularly when our behavior is based on fear.

Our fearful responses are usually the result of past hurts. What is yours? Look inside yourself to understand your reaction. Consider other choices that will create a new possibility. When you decide to face the underlying, original source of pain, you have an opportunity to heal and choose another way of looking at things. Being honest about our motivations is hard work.

Nursing Dance: **Your Three "Self's"**

Let me explain why you may not understand your own intentions or reactions, much less someone else's: We all want to look good, so we create an image of ourselves that we want the world to see.

Our words and actions originate from three levels of intention: our Masked Self, our Negative Self, and our Higher Self.

The view of ourselves that we want others to see is called our masked self. The sole mission of our masked self is to look good. From this part of ourselves, we befriend those who view us as a good person.

If someone doesn't assess us as good, we want to discredit or eliminate the individual from our circle of friends. This part of us is only interested in impressing everyone with our goodness.

Even if this only happens unconsciously, we don't really care about the impact on others. We only care about what's in it for us. You may think this is not how you react, but we can easily deceive ourselves regarding our motivations. So, don't discount this too soon.

The second part of our intent comes from our negative self, sometimes called our lower self. This part of us lashes out at others if we don't get the approval we want. From this part, we blow up at close friends or relatives who don't think we're great. If they don't give us what we want by maintaining this mirage, they'd better watch out.

I tell my friends that only my husband knows this part of me for sure.

Usually it is the people who are closest to us whom we attack when we don't like how they see us. From this lower part of us, we will attack anyone who doesn't maintain our vision of our masked image.

This behavior is probably the number one reason for the high divorce rate today, since the people who live with us twenty-four hours a day are most likely to see the good, the bad, and the ugly.

The third part of us is our higher self, which can accept imperfection in ourselves and others. From this more authentic part of us, we don't have to judge others or ourselves because we know and accept how difficult it is to overcome many of the perspectives we learned in childhood.

We realize that each of us has had difficulties and people who taught us to view life a certain way. We can accept and forgive the weaknesses in others when we accept and forgive our own.

A word of caution: If fear overcomes you, you will have difficulty staying in touch with your higher self. However, when you respond from your higher self, you are more likely to be clearer and get your point across. You will reduce the receiver's likelihood of resistance. Getting back in touch with your higher self when someone hurts you helps you to be objective and merciful and see new possibilities.

If you want to solve a problem, you need to respond from your higher self where your intention is open-minded, serene, and focused on resolution.

The way most of us handle challenges is to try to control the world to prevent feeling the old pain. Learning to accept whatever happens as a way to heal will allow you to go into the pain, understand its source, and become peaceful with it. Focus on what you can control: your response.

Nursing Dance: Finding the Solution

How can we be consistently accepting? *To increase your success with your partner in the nurse dance, take some time to understand what is creating your fear. Then bring yourself back to that part of you that wants to solve the problem instead of blaming someone for it.*

Take time to visualize being successful, happy, fulfilled, joyful, and any other possibility you would like to create before you proceed further.

Each time you replace your old way of being fearful and hurt with your new way of being lighthearted or loving, you feel the energy of your new possibility.

Think about all the things that created your strong endurance. You do not become resilient by seeking those situations that keep you sheltered and protected.

You become robust by learning to maneuver through all different circumstances and finding your sense of power and guidance from within.

If you find yourself feeling negative or drained after you do things for people, it is a sign that you are not acting out of your natural energy and your authentic or higher self.

Energies such as anger, frustration, anxiety, impatience, hurt feelings, complaining, righteousness, stubbornness, indifference, incompetence, laziness, lack of self-direction, negativity, helplessness, neediness, manipulation, blaming, and controlling provide indicators that you are acting out of some conditioned fear rather than out of your free spirit of giving.

As you come to grips with your true motivation, you may find yourself more in touch with the original source of your pain.

If you start to have resentment because of your difficult child-hood, begin to appreciate all the strength you've gained from the past situation. If it is difficult for you to feel loving toward some people in your life, find a way to view them as offering you an opportunity for growth. Use all the situations in your life as a way to identify your natural energy.

You can recognize the kind of energy you have difficulty being around without losing a peaceful feeling. Then you have an opportunity to behave differently and affect the situation permanently.

Though the process is not always simple to accomplish, it can be achieved if your foundation is sound and you are focused on creating something new. Knowing your gifts can help.

Nursing Dance: Know Your Gifts

When we are living consistent with our design, life becomes joyous. *Discover Your God-Given Gifts* by Don and Katie Fortune describes seven gifts based on the biblical reference in Romans 12:6 "Since we have gifts that differ according to the grace given to us, let us exercise them." The Fortunes identify the gifts as perceiving, exhorting (encouraging), serving, teaching, giving, administrating, and compassion. Though some level of each is in all of us, one gift is dominant and a second gift is very influential. Our gifts drive us and offer our greatest joy as we function within these innate tendencies. We experience ourselves more fully. Our flow from our natural source of energy contrasts the drain of forcing ourselves to be something we're not in the hopes of feeling external approval.

Our gifts are as distinctive and diverse as the ballroom dances. The gift of perceiving might be compared to a tango. The domi-nant walking movements of the tango have a dramatic powerful character. Movements are distinct, either slow and slithery, or sharp and cut short. American-style tango makes great use of open and alternate dance positions to further showcase tango's dramatic nature. Inspired perceivers tend to be bold, dynamic, intuitive, and morally clear. Perceivers feel compelled to speak up for causes and to warn others about pitfalls, making them courageous and direct. The greatest act of love for the perceiver is to risk everything to tell the truth. With pure confidence they make decisions about correct judgment and are very persuasive. Perceivers can have difficulty building friendships because of their blunt opinions. These people function from a perspective of decisively doing the right thing. They feel empowered by the improvement of an organization where their insights are applied. They like strong, secure leadership and open communication channels. They prefer an open culture where "telling it like it is" is embraced. When working with a perceiving person, communication can be enhanced by being direct and cutting to the chase. If you speak with conviction and take their intuition seriously, you will work best with them. To bring out the best in them, give them feedback about how their input affected your decision and don't overreact to the intensity of the conversation.

It may be suitable to compare the exhorter or encourager to the cha-cha. It's fun, energetic, sexy, flirtatious, and easily distinguished. The music is energetic and with a steady beat. The upbeat, exhorting person has an encouraging nature, loves to interact with people, and gets in tune quickly to relational and team dynamics. These people are verbal and pragmatic. The optimistic and growth-oriented exhorter encourages and challenges others to reach their potential. They are positive, accepting, and more interested in growth and personal progress than whether things are done exactly "right." Every situation becomes an opportunity for growth and change. Encouragers thrive on being helpful and seek to influence by persuasion. They hold a commonsense approach to problems because of their belief that they learn from life's experiences. When hurt or immature, exhorters can become overly dependent on the approval from other people. Under pressure, they can try to improve the situation by stretching the truth or seeing everything through an optimistic fantasy. They work best in flexible environments with relational opportunities. They like to process decisions verbally and having the ability to change things that aren't working.

To enhance your communication with exhorters, offer your full attention and warn them when you're interrupted. Build a relationship and give feedback so they know you've heard them. Exhorters need to work on issues with stretching the truth, being a know-it-all, and interrupting.

The server is like a foxtrot. Foxtrot is a smooth progressive dance, characterized by long, continuous flowing movements across the dance floor, offering casual and unhurried look. But there is more variety in foxtrot and, in some ways; it is the hardest dance to learn. Servers would rather do a job than delegate it. They are helpful, meticulous, practical, doers. They are present-oriented and have great dexterity. They tend to be selfless volunteers, even at their family's expense. They sense great joy doing a task and are energized by its completion. As a result, they like short-term projects and appreciation for their contributions. They are detail-oriented, neat, and want to do things right. They shy away from the limelight and projects that are mostly theoretical, social, or relational. They're great at meeting the needs of others, and show love by deeds and actions rather than words.

Servers function best in environments that have clear instructions and assistant roles. They like to be able to see the end of the project and get verbal praise. They need to know they are important, needed, and valued. To communicate best with servers, pay attention to their nonverbal cues that might indicate that they are not feeling comfortable or appreciated. Encourage them to express themselves and let them work while they're talking. These people need time to process new information. They can grow by allowing other people freedom not to serve others and by being aware of putting their family's needs before those of others. They also could benefit from maintaining their own energy when appreciation is lacking.

The administrator can measure up to the salsa, an exciting and inviting upbeat dance. It is anything but routine. Hot, spicy, and full of exotic Latin flavor, the salsa is true to its name, "saucy." The inspiring administrators are just as inviting and exciting. They are the vibrant natural leaders. With the ability to bring order out of chaos, they can express a vision that motivates others to get involved in long-term projects. They enjoy organizing people and projects. They like ongoing projects and see success as a group achievement. They are goal-oriented, value efficiency, and hate red tape. These people don't do well with routine, so they work well with servers who want a leader. They like to develop their own solutions and are determined catalysts for change. They want to know what the boundaries are and the lines of authority. Autonomy is important as well as the ability to pioneer new goals.

To communicate effectively with these people, be concise and avoid rambling. Be open to exploring different viewpoints. Be organized and value their time. They can benefit from being aware of their tendency to being driven and using people to get things done. They can sometimes have a hard shell, neglect routine tasks, and blur the boundaries between work and family.

The giver might be compared to the meringue, the easiest dance to learn. Surprisingly, it has not received wide recognition from the dancing public even though it is simple and gratifying. Generosity is the dance of the giver. The joyful giver is industrious, hospitable, and financially shrewd. These people have a knack for making money and making the best of what they have.

Givers love value and are great bargain seekers. They're practical and hard working and value excellence and integrity. They hate waste and want to make sure that any investments are handled with great care. They have a natural sense of what is needed and are very quick to react if someone tries to take advantage of them. If hurt or immature, they can be tightwads or selfish or they may take care only of themselves. The best environment for a giver is one with high standards and integrity that strives for excellence. These people are at their best when they are close to people whose needs they know. They want to make a difference, and they have a wonderful gift of seeing and developing ways to be more economical.

If you want to communicate well with givers, have regular meetings to update them on progress and follow through on your agreements. Show value for them and their contribution. Ask them for their suggestions, which are founded in common sense. Administrators could improve by looking for ways to give without conditions attached. They may need to keep their work in balance and become more predictable. In some cases, growth would come from not spoiling their children and grandchildren or from just allowing other people to not give.

The gift of the teacher is best compared to the waltz, a smooth progressive dance characterized by long, flowing movements, continuous turns, and rise and falls. Graceful and elegant waltz dancers glide around the floor almost effortlessly. The expressive quality of the music often invites very powerful and dynamic movement from dancers.

Teachers are highly skilled in their area of interest. Naturally inquisitive and analytical, they have a systematic approach to learning and are generally even-tempered and objective. They are guided by their principles. Teachers are thinkers and love research. They can be walking encyclopedias on a particular subject and would never take the word of someone without researching the source. They love to share their knowledge with others and like to be with intellectually stimulating friends. They can be resistant to change and prone to getting distracted with trivial data pursuits. They could benefit from working on their relationship skills and becoming more focused and practical. Teachers want to understand how a system works and be able to create new systems of information. They like having the opportunity to learn new things.

The compassionate person might be most like the gentle rumba, an emotional dance with rolling turns, soft strutting, and seductive motion. Guitar and piano keep a steady beat and fill in the harmony. A singer or instrumental soloist usually takes the melody.

The compassionate person feels deep emotions. These are caring, sensitive, self-sacrificing, empathetic, and thoughtful people. They don't function well in high-pressure environments and can benefit from frequent, positive encouragement. They love to be in contact with other people and will shy away from tough decisions. Be gentle when confronting or challenging compassionate people. Their affectionate expressions might be misinterpreted by the opposite sex. They want their relationships with others to run smoothly and to give positive encouragement. The compassionate person is generally cheerful, sincere, and great at celebrating everyone's victories. When in the pits, these people can be indecisive, inconsistent, and overly sensitive. Because others easily hurt them, they frequently need healing from past hurts to lead full lives.

Nurses dispense compassion on a regular basis and sometimes grow weary of feeling and delivering it. We may even entertain fantasies of never having to show empathy or compassion again. We all know a least one nurse who used to be competent and caring, and then something changed. She began to complain, hate her job, and make everyone around her miserable. These are symptoms of compassion fatigue. She is the nurse none of us want to become.

Most professionals believe this condition is the result of traumatic stress from exposure to victims of physical or emotional trauma. The nursing profession is at high risk of compassion fatigue because of our deep, caring commitment to our hurting patients. We need to be aware of the risk of compassion fatigue and make plans for prevention, self-care, and peer support.

Knowing our vulnerability is the first step. If we are proactive and self-caring, prevent the loss of wonderful assets and the magnificent gift of compassion that nurses bring to people in need. We can start by looking for ways we can receive every time we give. Receiving should be a big part of the incentive for giving. When we feel that we are giving beyond our capacity, we must make some adjustment. This requires being more nurturing toward ourselves and sometimes making changes in our physical surroundings.

A Nurse's Story

I watched my mother, who was a nurse who worked private-duty nights to be with us after school. She usually picked up cases around the holidays and before school started so that she would have the extra money to take care of the added expenses. When everyone came over for Thanksgiving dinner, I remember her complaining that no one helped her clean up. She wanted to have both families at her home so she could see and please everyone. These get-togethers were some of my favorite memories. Eventually, she became a compassion fatigue victim and stopped doing anything for anyone. Even sadder, she didn't want anyone to do anything for her.

Looking back, my mother wasn't free to do what she wanted because of her desire to please others. She was so focused outside and knew nothing about what was going on inside herself. If my dad wanted her to go somewhere and she didn't want to go, he was criti-

cal. *When eventually she became depressed, we lost the wonderful person who wanted to bring everyone together.*

Depression is really the state of suppressed feelings. It can make us feel hopeless, afraid, alone, and convinced that things will never get better. It's like a black curtain of despair coming down over a person's life. Many depressed people have no energy and can't concentrate; others feel irritable all the time for no apparent reason. Many take medication for these responses, yet never really get to the bottom of the issue. To prevent this response to life, we must build our personal awareness. Knowledge about our individual values provides another key to unlock the door to our consciousness.

Nursing Dance: **Know Your Values**

Personal values offer a clear picture of what we want. If we are able to create an environment that we find valuable, we will experience contentment. Otherwise, we become frustrated and resentful without knowing why. Understanding is the first step to improving our situation. Since values drive us, becoming acquainted with them allows us to truly clarify who we are.

Identifying your values in ten specific aspects of your life will serve to open your eyes to your reality. Until you spend time examining what you want, you will have no idea what you're striving toward and why. You may be frustrated with no explanation. For example, the definition of financial stability can vary significantly. One person may want luxury cars while another wants simplicity and enough to give to others. These differences can result in a magnitude of problems if they are not recognized and defined.

Values are lifelong wishes. We may be unaware of our need to control people and situations that results from our desire to have things a certain way.

A Nurse's Story

I value mutual support and fun in my family. I grew up in a family with competition for scarce resources. Rivalry may be good in sports, but it didn't make for a peaceful home. My parents were so engrossed in their own warfare that they had little time to help their six daughters feel special. It was strange to me that my sisters weren't affected the same way I was. Until I realized that my value was getting and giving support, I had no idea why I was so disappointed with my family. I was driven to fix them and create the family I thought we should be. It never occurred to me to accept the disparity until I fully recognized our differences. On an unconscious level, I was giving what I wanted to get and wondering why they wouldn't give it back.

Over the years, I became more and more resentful, to the point of getting angry when they called for encouragement. I felt used and unappreciated. I was unaware that I wanted something from them that I wasn't getting. As part of my personal coaching, I was guided to identify my values. This exploration was eye-opening since I was teaching people how to treat me. Thinking that everyone knew how families should treat each other, I assumed they were too wounded to do anything different. In reality, I didn't know what they valued. I had no contact with my feelings until my anger started rearing its ugly head.

To know yourself, know what you value. You probably have different values from many people you know. It may feel scary to discover this difference with the people you are closest to, such as your spouse and siblings. However, it is a great starting point for insight.

Knowing our values is a wonderful gift for our marriage and workplace. How many of you were taught to dissect and understand your values? Every one of us thinks life should be a certain way. What we don't realize is that everyone else we meet doesn't perceive life the same way. We are unknowingly egocentric. We truly believe everyone thinks like us. We think that the fact that someone else is not doing things the way we would is because they are being difficult. All of our differences have the same foundation.

Our range of diversity originates in what we cherish. Values are central to our expectations. Until we identify our distinctive core beliefs, they may continue to influence situations negatively below our awareness. Disconnection will occur without comprehension. Being aware of what is important to us brings clarity, self-expression, and focus. We have the opportunity to share our understanding with the people we care about. Even more importantly, we are able to recognize what disturbs us about situations that arise. We can then consciously choose to alter, avoid, or accept what is happening.

There are ten fundamental areas of your life where exploration is worthwhile. Your spiritual life, marital or single life, family and children, work, church/ministry, financial, physical, personal development, social, and recreation and hobbies all are key to creating contentment in your world. Awareness gives perspective into direction and motivation.

Your spiritual life, including your personal relationship with God and your personal or family worship practices, has a powerful effect on you. Your spiritual life is very private and deliberating about what you want is fruitful, especially knowing when you're not getting it.

Your marriage or single life reveals volumes about your level of fulfillment with your place in the world. It includes your ability to make choices in mates, your feelings about relationships, and your role you play with your spouse. Single life relates to roommates, dating or lack of dating, and personal standards for intimate relationships.

Your family and children relationships involve dealing with schooling, discipline, and the choice of fun activities. It is also comprised of relationships with your extended family, including grandchildren, siblings, ill parents, and grandparents. You determine how much you want to keep in touch and whether you want to be involved in family gatherings.

When looking at your work life, think about your professional relationships and entrepreneurial activities. Determine what characteristics you want in your job.

Your personal development requirements are another area to ascertain. Ask yourself how you want to exercise your intellect and build skills. Determine the amount of reading, formal education, workshops and conferences in which you want to engage. Ask yourself if you want to learn to play an instrument, write, paint, or learn a language.

Consider what level of church or spiritual involvement would best suit you. Does belonging to a church seem important? How vital is being involved in small groups, belonging to a committee, having a leadership role, or working on a service project?

Another area to review is your financial requirements. Evaluate feelings about finances in general and then budgeting and recordkeeping. Look at areas such as retirement planning and investments. Include giving and tithing. Think about whether you're taking good care of the possessions you have.

Next, discover your physical care desires and determine how you want to take care of your body. Nutrition, eating habits, dieting habits, exercise, medical care, and stress management would be included here.

Assess your social activities and friendships. Is being involved in your community important? Your inclination to join social clubs, the school board, PTA; coach a sport; or belong to a political organization would be evaluated here.

Concerning recreation and hobbies identify how you relax. Taking vacations, having holiday gatherings, going on outings, having hobbies, going out to dinner, giving and attending parties, and playing sports would be included in this area.

Whether we realize it or not, our values affect our decisions and relationships. When evaluating your values, give yourself plenty of time to explore, because the recognition process is not always straightforward. Some of you may have unknowingly given up wishing and wanting things because you didn't receive the things you wanted in childhood. You have to know what you want before you can ask for it. Otherwise, you are unconsciously undermining your own happiness.

Take the time to look at these ten areas to determine what your life would look like if you had what you wanted. Determine what is important to you in each category. Evaluate how far away you are from what you want. Then start discovering ways to get from point A, what you have, to point B, what you want.

Ask yourself where you feel passionate, where you would spend your time and money, what you would be willing to sacrifice for, and why would you sacrifice for it. Wonder about what makes you distinctive and stand out from others. Examine what gets you excited. Recognize what gets you on your soapbox. Identify what you find yourself talking about all the time.

Figure out why you care about the things you care about. These answers will tell you what makes you unique, which will help you identify your soul position here on earth. Once you know what excites you, you're ready to understand what's underlying your choices. Our choices drive our life and have the power to transform us.

Nursing Dance: **The Power of Choice**

Once you become unemotional and act from your calm, clear center, the action you take can create any way of being that you choose.

If someone is trying to intimidate, threaten, or control you, imagine him or her as one inch tall. If people are angry or aggressive, picture them as small children throwing tantrums because they are coming from their little selves and not their higher selves.

Fighting with them brings you down to their level. Staying calm and centered will allow you to become more effective in any situation. Before and after you enter any new place, be aware of your own energy so that you can evaluate whether you are being affected by the energy of that place.

As nurses, we are sensitive to the feelings and needs of others. This is a gift, unless it is used for the purpose of being accepted by others rather than as a calling. Being aware of your own energy will give you a frame of reference that allows you to get in touch with your motivation.

It takes work to understand what is happening within us and permanently transform the situation to a new possibility, so be patient yet relentless. Your nurse dance is joyful when you make the effort and stay grounded and flexible.

Nursing Dance: **Stay Grounded and Flexible**

Just as my instructor told me to bend my knees to stay grounded and flexible, we nurses need to stay grounded and flexible within our convictions. Dancers hold their abdomen in and keep their chest high while imagining a string holding them suspended. As nurses, we hold assurance in and keep our attitude high and are suspended by our authentic identity. In so doing, we can respond to any situation through our natural loving and accepting energy.

Dancers start by getting the right frame and then learn to maintain it. In nursing, we also need to start with establishing the right frame of reference and then maintain it in whatever may come our way.

Now that you know how to establish your frame, let us move on and learn to maintain it.

Questions to Explore

1. What are your values in the following areas: social life, work life, family life, personal development, marriage/single life, spiritual/church life, physical fitness, recreational/hobbies?

2. In what areas of your personal or professional life do you fear taking a stand?

3. Where do you want to be in a year (or five years)? What do you see yourself doing?

4. What is stopping you from moving forward?

5. If you saw someone else in your situation, what would you tell him or her?

III.

Maintain Your Frame

*I would not know what the spirit of a philosopher
might wish more to be than a good dancer.*
Friedrich Nietzsche (1844-1900)

I was locked in place like a deer in headlights when my instructor began to speak.

"Start the dance by walking back with your right leg and pushing off with your left foot. Glide your right foot back so that your toe touches the floor first while you move your leg from the hip maintaining the bend in your knee."

Not sure how I could do all that at once, I moved my right leg back. My head was full of instructions and my body stiff and resistant. My elbows dropped as I moved and after my right leg was back, I became immobilized again as if the concept of moving my left leg was totally foreign. With my instructor's encouragement, I moved my other leg and then continued walking the length of the room. Each step gave me a little more confidence, and then it was time to walk backward while turning.

When I accidentally straightened my legs or dropped the lift in my upper body, I began to lose my sense of balance.

Learning something new demands great concentration to details. My dance lesson taught me that movement of any kind requires motivation. We all have the choice to embrace a new possibility or stay stuck right where we are.

How would your life be
if you saw all situations as opportunities for growth
and used every circumstance as an opening to learn
something new about you?

As nurses, our lives are never dull. We have more challenges than we know what to do with on any given day. If we look at challenges as something to learn from rather than frustrations, we move beyond them with energy and ease. We can ask for what we want and create environments that serve us as well as others.

One nurse started working in a new area where no one socialized. At her last place, people would get together after work and held a Christmas party. Her first thought was to adjust to the new culture. After exploring her wish a little further, she decided to take responsibility for starting something new. She asked a few people if they would be interested and before she knew it, they were going out after work twice a month. She organized the first Christmas party with her nurse manager's encouragement. The doctor attended and paid for everyone's first drink.

Another nurse was a constant complainer. Her colleagues were so tired and frustrated with her that they decided to bring it to her attention. To their surprise, she had no idea how she was coming across and welcomed their suggestion of keeping a list of things for which she was grateful. She decided to make a poster and have people add to the list until the poster was full. The camaraderie in the department grew and people started helping each other get their work done. She remembered the day her peer told her she was a "perpetual downer." The group began to fix the little annoyances in the department and made it a much more joyous place to work.

You have every right to have the kind of job and work environment you enjoy. However, you may have to move past wishing someone else would make it happen and take action.

Nursing Dance: **Take Action**

Doing nothing is a choice, and it has consequences. Motivation is the foundation of our choices. Our first step is hard, often not pretty, and yet required to advance. When our core is centered and balanced, we progress and keep upright. The way to find our center is to feel secure in who we are.

> ## We can be
> ## a grand and glorious ship
> ## that never leaves the harbor.

Most people stay where they are until the pain of remaining is greater than the fear of change.

When we take the time to know our values and motivation, we are able to maintain the balance and flexibility needed to smoothly glide through life's dance.

There is always some fear linked with doing something new. In the words of Dale Carnegie, "Confidence comes from walking through fear." Facing our fear head on allows us to walk through it. Fear can prevent us from being authentic. Because of fear, we often don't accomplish what we want.

We don't fix difficulties if we are always sidestepping the real issue. The fear is not coming from the outside world, but from our inner dialogue.

We respond to the outside world based on our internal beliefs. If we think things outside of us must change if we are to be happy, we will always be looking for happiness. If we think other people need to change to create a safer environment, we will be trapped in a world of fear and trepidation.

Taking action and asking for what we want is easier for some because of behavioral type. We are not all created the same. However, we all can have what we want if we accept the need for development of some behaviors that just don't come naturally. Insight into our behavioral type and motivation can help.

Nursing Dance: **Know your Type**

Understand that we all want to have our needs met and to eliminate whatever we are afraid of. Until you know what drives you, you will be motivated to act out of fear rather than desire.

There are four specific ways in which you are motivated and deal with fear. Challenge, power, and authority motivate some of you. You fear loss of control and being taken advantage of. You can be all about business and direct answers, acting confident and bold. Unaware of your own fear, you can exhibit an impatient lack of concern for others. Criticizing some of these qualities is easy. Yet in reality, these are very often good leadership qualities if coupled with the emotional intelligence that allows you to manage fears, be realistic, and respect other people's needs.

This is you if you feel compelled to tell everyone what to do and how to do it—and if you don't have much concern for how others take your advice and direction. You think you are right, and if people have a problem with you, that is their problem.

Many of you are motivated by social recognition, group activities, and relationships. You are enthusiastic, charming, and sociable. You generally fear social rejection, disapproval, and

loss of influence. Your limitations are impulsiveness, disorgani-
zation, and lack of follow-through.

Here, emotional intellect needs to be utilized to think
through your actions and reduce impulsiveness and disorgani-
zation. Care must be taken to commit only to what you will
follow through on. Establishing internal security allows you to
handle whatever happens and reduces your fear of losing influence and the need for constant approval.

This is you if you are the one who always wants to get the
party started. You want each staff meeting to be fun and social
as well as informative. You may be the one to set up occasions
to meet up with other staff member after work and organize the
Christmas party or birthday celebrations.

An environment that has infrequent change, stability, sincere appreciation, and cooperation motivates some of you. You
are patient, calm, stable, methodical, and team players as long
as everything is going well. However, you fear a loss of stability,
the unknown, change, and unpredictability. In relationships,
you tend to be overly willing to give and address your needs
last. Benefit will be derived from the ability to self-soothe as you
recognize and accept that things are constantly changing. You
should identify your needs and fulfill them.

You know this is you if you are very appreciative of the person who creates the balance of work and social environment on
the nursing unit. You like the social aspect of your job and are
disappointed if that is not part of the work milieu. You might
work extra hours just so people are happy with you and conflict
on the unit is reduced.

Many of you are motivated by having clearly defined performance expectations with quality and accuracy valued. You
are cautious, precise, diplomatic, and restrained in behavior.
However, you fear criticism of your work and dislike slipshod
methods. At times you are limited by being overly critical of

others and yourself. You tend to be indecisive because of your desire to collect and analyze data.

For you, being aware of and appreciating your own drive for quality is helpful. To view people's opinions of your work as an opportunity for improvement and even more success is helpful. Benefit will occur when you lighten up on yourself and others by seeing the gift in an expanded perspective. Since perfection is not a possible destination, you must start celebrating progress.

You know this is you if you are concerned when things change because it reduces your ability to sustain high quality. You like things to stay consistent because you know you can maintain patient safety and excellent care. You become frustrated if others don't see the importance of maintaining quality above all else.

The more you know yourself and embrace your fears, strengths, and weaknesses, the better every experience will feel. Your success increases your ability to positively interpret and respond to situations with authenticity. A constant barrage of things happens outside your direct control. Accepting others in your home and work environment allows joy to be experienced. These things increase flexibility just as the dance frame does. As you recognize your style and the styles of others, you can adapt as needed. Learning to find your footing helps you create what you really want. No one is purely one style. You can take an assessment to identify your preference at www. SaveTheFirstDanceForYou.com

Once we understand our type, the next area to examine is our defenses. We develop defenses based on our fears. Once we understand how we defend ourselves, we can create something to serve our needs effectively.

Nursing Dance: **Know Your Defense Mechanisms**

Our defense mechanisms can be an unconscious means of protecting us from unpleasant emotions. When we face a difficult or anxiety-producing situation, we may engage in intellectual analysis of the events and our defenses may be triggered to reduce the associated tension. Defense mechanisms are a means to reduce apprehension by distancing, transforming, or falsifying our circumstances. They reduce our anxiety and allow us to cope with whatever we're facing.

Two positive defense mechanisms are affiliating with others and humor. It is helpful to connect with other people and share our problems or difficulties without trying to make someone else responsible for them. Relationships are beneficial for both help and support. Humor, not sarcasm that is indirect anger, is another constructive means of coping with worry. We can release tension by noticing amusing or ironic aspects of a situation. Persons who successfully use humor have the capacity to stand outside themselves and observe and comment on the events that affect others and themselves. This allows them to tolerate the situation while still focusing on what is happening.

Less useful defense mechanisms protect us from being consciously aware of a thought or feeling that we cannot tolerate. These defenses only allow the unconscious thought or feeling to be expressed indirectly in a disguised form. Let's say you are angry with your nurse manager because she is very critical of you. Here's how John Suler of Rider University identifies for his clinical psychology students the various defenses might hide and/or transform that anger:

Denial: You completely reject the thought or feeling. "I'm not angry with her!"

Suppression: You are vaguely aware of the thought or feeling, but try to hide it. "I'm going to try to be nice to her."

Reaction Formation: You turn the feeling into its opposite. "I think she's really great!"

Projection: You think someone else has your thought or feeling. "That nurse manager hates me." "That other nurse hates the nurse manager."

Displacement: You redirect your feelings to another target. "I hate that secretary."

Rationalization: You come up with various explanations to justify the situation while denying your feelings. "She's so critical because she's trying to help us do our best."

Intellectualization: A type of rationalization, only more intellectualized. "This situation reminds me of how Nietzsche said that anger is ontological despair."

Undoing: You try to reverse or undo your feeling by doing something that indicates the opposite feeling. It may be an "apology" for the feeling you find unacceptable within yourself. "I think I'll give that nurse manager a gift."

Isolation of Affect: You "think" the feeling but don't really feel it. "I guess I'm angry with her, sort of."

Regression: You revert to an old, usually immature behavior to ventilate your feeling. "Let's laugh, and have side conversations at staff meetings!"

Sublimation: You redirect the feeling into a socially productive activity. "I'm going to write a poem about anger."

Defenses may hide any of a variety of thoughts or feelings: anger, fear, sadness, depression, greed, envy, competitiveness, love, passion, admiration, criticalness, dependency, selfishness, grandiosity, helplessness. The more we can become aware of how we defend against our authentic feelings, the more likely we will be able to break the cycle of unhealthy defenses. It is much more important to know what we think and feel before making a conscious choice about how to handle the situation.

According to Suler, a beneficial way to get defense mechanisms out in the open is to do some role-playing. It's worthwhile to develop a role-play that you can perform at the next staff meeting. Have people demonstrate several defense mechanisms. Try to give everyone a part to play. Good role-plays usually spend a minute or so to develop the scene, the characters, and the situation at hand. At that point, start to introduce the defenses into the scene. The whole role-play should last about three to five minutes. After you finish the scene, the staff will try to guess which defense mechanisms you were demonstrating. Our goal should always be to break through our own denial. Recognition is the first step to recover our authentic self.

Nursing Dance: Being Authentic

Dancers can imagine a string lifting them up into their proper dance frame. As nurses, we can imagine a force lifting us up to access our true/authentic self. It's your connection with your authentic self and your intention to accept what you cannot change that strengthens you and allows you to let go of power struggles.

Your recognition and courage to change what you can change will lift you and allow you to respond positively. Remember that you can only transform your response to the world through your way of being. Your goal is to gain the wisdom to know the difference between what you can control and what you can't.

You can never change people, places, and things in your life. You can only transform your response to the outside world by seeing yourself clearly and truly accepting how you are being. If you're being resistant or hurt, you will continually see people as pushing and hurting you. Being totally honest gives you access to your power and control to transform the situation.

If you will take the time to notice that you are being resistant, resentful, defensive, or critical in a situation, you can then identify what you need. Maybe you identify that you need acceptance, affirmation, freedom, or approval. You can then be transformed by being accepting, affirming, loving, or approving. Your can actually feel yourself being lifted up with this new way of being. Being real and authentic with yourself can provide what you need.

You can then stop doing things you don't want to do and start accepting the feelings that come up. You can observe your feelings and understand why you are so driven to keep your actions going. Only then are you capable of facing the conflict arising from within and exist outside of you.

Nursing Dance: Facing Conflict

I think it's easy to say that none of you really want to deal with conflict. You would like others to create a milieu that reduces the amount of your conflict. If you shift this goal to learning about how you respond to other people, you can alter your internal as well as the external struggle. Conflict can be viewed as a state that exposes your internal process. The challenges of the outside world help reveal what already exists inside you. If you take the time to understand and own what is being awakened inside you, you can embrace your uniqueness.

Once you fully accept yourself, no one will create the feeling of conflict and disapproval within you.

When you react to something, ask yourself what that touched within. Find your wound and spend time with yourself to feel your own pain. The only way to heal is to own your wounding and pain. That doesn't mean you caused it. It just means it's your personal experience. You can spend so much time running away from your own feelings and blaming the people around you for producing those feelings that you forget or never realize that you own your feelings. Your feelings are an expression of you. The other person only tapped into them. Other people do not cause your feelings. Accepting this fact makes the real distinction.

Knowing our feelings come from within give us an opportunity to heal old wounds.

Nursing Dance: **Healing Old Wounds**

All of us have experienced things in childhood that were too much to handle emotionally. Yes, some have been victims of horrid abuse, but this is not a requirement for wounds to occur. A parent who didn't give us something that seemed really important can wound us. A friend's rejection can be enough of a reason to bury painful feelings associated with it. We can have conflict avoidance characteristics for many reasons. Facing the truth will liberate you. Facing resistance and overcoming it will free you from the bonds of conflict fear.

Facing the reality about our fears from childhood is the first step. We are often raised to focus on external approval. We want our parents to be happy with us. Most parents are not so enlightened that they realize that resistance from a child should be embraced as a statement of self. Most of us didn't have parents who were aware of the need for us to know ourselves and to be ourselves. They just wanted us to be acceptable in society. They often wanted us to make them feel proud. In so doing, however unintentional, they primed us to feel good about ourselves only when others approve of us.

Most don't realize that the motivation behind the compulsive need for approval. We fear someone becoming angry with us. We can't risk being rejected. Trust and fear are on opposite sides of the spectrum. When we see the other person as more powerful, or we see ourselves losing control, we fear what might happen.

In our desire for peace and harmony, approval seekers must be hyper vigilant about avoiding conflict. It may be hard to recognize that we have a lack of trust inside ourselves. We may think we are just doing the right thing. When we do acknowledge our lack of trust, we are really saying we don't trust *our response* to the people around us. It is a statement about us, not just the environment. Only by looking directly at the source of our fear can we let go of it and experience being trusting. Our thoughts give us insight into our fear.

Nursing Dance: **Know Your Thoughts**

As John Locke said, "The actions of men are the best interpreters of their thoughts." Let's step back and consider two responses to fear.

Those with a high drive to control the environment to stay safe tend to be more assertive and extroverted. They are more likely to have an outward response to stress and fight rather than run. They are more ready to communicate, faster paced, more forceful, and more aggressive as well as more decisive and impatient.

In contrast, those individuals who have more of a tendency to adapt to stay safe are less assertive and more introverted. They are hesitant to communicate, slower paced, soft-spoken, more deliberate, thoughtful, and patient.

We also can be divided into two groups based on whether we are task or relationship-oriented. The task-oriented group is reserved, filled with facts, restrained, distant, and disciplined. The relationship-oriented group is relaxed, playful, outgoing, easier to get to know, and carefree.

Though certainly not 100 percent, nurses tend to be relationship-oriented adapters. We will let other people do things and say things we don't like, then lick our wounds in silence or complain to uninvolved coworkers. We fear making things worse by speaking up. Sometimes we lash out at some safe target, accomplishing nothing worthwhile. We are afraid to feel our anger even when it is legitimate. We fear dealing with other people's anger.

We don't want to feel the sadness associated with disconnecting from people we care about. We want to avoid feeling old hurts from childhood. However, protecting ourselves from old pain compels us to keep ourselves completely numb or running from the pain.

We become workaholics, alcoholics, overeaters, and compulsive meddlers or pleasers just to keep ourselves from feeling our pain. We resent pushing ourselves down in this way, even if we are unaware of it, and the pressure of anger builds and festers. This can unknowingly result in manipulative or passive-aggressive behavior.

This is coupled with the fact that most physicians have a high drive to control the environment and task orientation. Their aggressive style is a perfect setup to make it tremendously difficult for nurses to take action.

In reality, the most effective way to handle conflict is to candidly express our issues without judgment. Recognize you own your pain and that only you can deal with it effectively. Owning and accepting your feelings is the beginning of creating a new experience. Too many of us grew up seeing or experiencing physical or verbal abuse. The fear of reliving it is deep. Love and hate for the abuser is very confusing. We come out of those situations thinking we controlled the environment by complying or avoiding direct conflict.

We try to keep everything calm within ourselves while feeling like failures when we are unsuccessful at maintaining a peaceful atmosphere. We believe this kept us safe as children, and we try to keep ourselves safe as adults.

If we don't examine our behavior and our motivation before we move forward, others will always be able to knock us off-balance. Our lack of grounding and stability exists because we are intertwined with the people around us.

We need to know ourselves and accept and value our contribution. We need to stand strong and steady on our own, or we will always be dependent on others to stabilize us, leaving us at their mercy. Just as the dancer starts alone, moving in all directions, so must you learn to be strong alone? We often go along because we fear the loss of approval, and it's important to know that doing this comes at a cost.

Nursing Dance: The Cost of Compliance

What may be even less evident is the resentment of maintaining this act of compliance. The adapter and controller inevitably become aggrieved. Questions begin to arise. Why doesn't anyone think about me? Why doesn't anybody listen to me? Why am I always taking care of everyone else and they don't return the favor? Maybe a pattern of giving and pulling back begins to happen. You do for others. They don't show appreciation for what you do. You get angry and stay away for a while. Next, you feel guilty and come back into the picture.

Maybe you also try to get others to see what they need to do to help you feel better. They show some form of rejection, and the cycle begins again. If it's happening with multiple people, you are constantly on the outs with someone and in turmoil about what to do. Continuously trying to adapt or control the outside world and running from our greatest fears is exhausting.

We think it's about other people rather than looking at the source—feeling unloved as a child. We want to know who we are without the obligation of pleasing others. When we don't receive love as a child, we erect an armor of defenses to protect ourselves against feeling unlovable. As a result, we are cut off from our ability to receive love.

In reality, the only way to be able to accept love is to face and acknowledge our fear of rejection and being hurt. Our parents may have loved us, though not in the way we wanted. It is not about what actually happened. It is about how we interpreted it. We create our own story about our life.

We are afraid of people's negative response because we don't want to touch the deep feeling of rejection we felt when we didn't get the love that should have been so natural. Feeling unloved from outside ourselves, we internalize the rejection. We don't love and appreciate ourselves. So, we really can't give or receive love.

I don't know any conscious people who had a perfect childhood. I say conscious people because there are people who will say they had a perfect childhood, but you can sense their unacknowledged resentment. This is not to say that everyone had a terrible childhood. It is only to say that all of us have been wounded in some way. People may act fearless and deny anger, but their life shows evidence of something else. It may be a feeling of stress, low energy, or being unfulfilled.

We human beings have a wonderful ability to use projection and transference to hide our real feelings. Projection is a powerful defense against personal unpleasantness. If our ego or lower self wants to stay in denial, we make the problem be about someone else. If we make them bad, we can be good. Unfortunately, this continuous cycle never solves the problems or results in the peace. Taking the time to examine what is really going on can release you from bondage of your unconscious mind.

Nursing Dance: Living an Examined Life

The following Chinese proverb says so much about the quest for self-awareness and wisdom. "He who knows not, and knows not that he knows not, is a fool–shun him. He who knows not, and knows that he knows not is ignorant–teach him. He who knows, and knows not that he knows, is asleep–wake him. But, he who knows, and knows he knows is a wise man–follow him." In the Bible, Proverbs 14:16 tells us, "The wise man is cautious and shuns evil; the fool is reckless and sure of himself."

Let's look at living an examined life. The first statement, "He who knows not, and knows not that he knows not, is a fool–shun him," is an example of unconscious incompetence, a

potentially dangerous position. If you spend too much time trying to convert these people, you will not only be wasting your
time, but you will also be dragged through the mud with them.
Sometimes life can shock an unconsciously incompetent person
into reality. They usually read a book such as this, hoping to fix
someone else.

When you realize that you have total control over your own
experience, there is great power in that. The unskilled driver
who gets confidently behind the wheel can cause havoc on the
road until he searches for needed guidance.

The second statement, "He who knows not, and knows that
he knows not is ignorant–teach him," describes individuals who
are at least conscious of their incompetence. These people see
their deficit and are hungry for knowledge. Anyone who is willing can learn. One of our operating room technicians had the
toughest time learning to scrub. I knew he wanted to succeed
and gave him the time and help to do so. If you are open and
willing, you can find the knowledge and skills you want and
need.

The third line of the proverb, "He who knows, and knows
not that he knows, is asleep—wake him," is an example of being
unconsciously competent. We often do things because we've
always done them and we become unconscious about the how
and the why. If you're an experienced nurse, you don't have to
think about how to perform an assessment or to use the nursing process. It is second nature. However, if you want to teach
these skills to someone else, you must become conscious of the
steps.

The last statement, "he who knows, and knows he knows,
is a wise man—follow him," is about conscious competence.
The consciously competent teacher is totally aware of the steps
required to accomplish a task. Becoming conscious of the details
is essential if you want to develop a new skill. When you want

to learn how to create a better experience for yourself, you must recognize your own style and patterns before you are able to create an environment in which you love to live and work.

A Nurse's Story

I was in a counseling setting with my husband when the counselor was trying to help us see one of our patterns. I was feeling very distant and afraid of my husband at the time. The counselor suggested that we stand, imagining a line down the center of the room that we couldn't cross. I stood far behind the line with my arms crossed for a fairly long period of time. My husband paced far behind the line on the other side of the room. He came to the edge of the line once and stood there for a short time and then went back to pacing. I eventually came to the edge of the line because I began feeling guilty that I didn't meet him there earlier, but he had waited such a short time. I stood there waiting.

It seemed like forever before he returned to his side of the line. I was so frustrated by the time he came that I gave him a little smack, hugged him, and began to cry very deeply for a long time. Much later, I recognized this pattern in real life. I would withdraw from people who hurt me and then feel guilty, move closer, but get angry when they came close. I would want to process the hurt. They would often be defensive. The cycle would start again. I was able to break the cycle when I saw how I created it.

A Nurse's Story

When I didn't feel loved, I responded by being hurt and isolating myself. I began to see the same pattern in other key relationships. My hurt was so great that I couldn't tolerate touching it. I feared I wouldn't be able to stop hurting if I started. I kept trying to keep everyone else happy, even though that is totally impossible. I didn't want to hurt, so I resisted consciousness of my pain and pattern. I was petrified by my childhood fear, so I tried to stay in control. I didn't want to feel my sadness or my anger.

Eventually, my feelings became so overwhelming that I started to crumble to the point of collapse. Feeling sorry for myself seemed unproductive unless I accepted it as a part of the process. I didn't see the pattern until I totally accepted responsibility for my feelings. Life got better when I stopped blaming other people and "owned my own experience," in the words of Dr. Phil McGraw. For the first time in my life, I became accountable for what I was creating.

During the withdrawn time, I was nonproductive. I just kept cycling through forcing myself to do something, so I didn't feel my own perceived badness. I wasn't honest. I was a fraud and that angered me, yet it all seemed so normal. My friends were frauds, too. Doing what needed to be done because we could and/or should.

A Nurse's Story

I decided whether to do something by answering three questions. First, did it need to be done? Second, could I do it? Third, could I be successful? I never considered whether I wanted to do it. I had pushed myself to do things all my life because they needed to be done. And I could do them. Therefore, they should be done. It was too scary to stop doing. What would people think if I changed? So I continued until I just didn't want to do anything except what gave me pleasure. I wanted to stop being around people who complained or made me feel bad.

I came to realize that I had created a world that wasn't fun. My friends were just as unhappy and kept cycling through their circle of unhappiness. I thought to myself, "I want new friends." What I really wanted was a new outlook with an attitude that didn't include the fear of being myself. I realized that the fear was locked inside of me and if I wanted to leave the prison I had created, I would have to honor who I was and face my fear and move beyond it.

The only reason to examine your life is to get to know who you are and honor yourself. To look at yourself as if there is something wrong only undermines who you are and what you bring to the world.

Nursing Dance: **Honor Who You Are**

Being sensitive to your emotions gives you insight into the state of your spirit. When your spirit is not being nurtured and honored, you will have negative emotional reactions. By letting go of the external focus, you can become aware of your internal process. Some feelings, like anger, may have been suppressed for so long that it's difficult to bring them to the surface. *Instead of medicating away your emotional or physical pain, spend quiet time asking for insight into your pain to assist in raising your consciousness. When you receive awareness about yourself and how you respond to others, trust it. Try to understand what the awareness is telling you about how well your life is working for you. You don't have to act on your awareness right away; recognize that feelings are temporary. No situation, feeling, or thought is constant. You cycle through the same patterns, so begin raising your consciousness and notice your patterns without judging them as good or bad. Own your feelings because your feelings are a window to your spirit.*

The truth is that you can't motivate yourself or other people. As you become aware of what is driving you, differentiate between what is natural and energy giving vs. what is learned, fear-based, and energy draining. You can create environments that inspire by understanding yourself first and then the others in the environment. People are wired differently; situations will bring out different behaviors based on awareness and unhealed wounds. The best thing you can do to create the kind of place where you love to live, work, or be is to identify what motivates you. If you want to create a stirring environment for others, get to know what stimulates them. A win-win

*environment where we live and work can be established by becoming
balanced, flexible, and consciously competent of the steps.*

Once you've acknowledged and honored who you are, you
can proactively develop a supportive culture for others.

Nursing Dance: **Consciously Develop the Culture**

Cultures develop with or without conscious involvement.
Family members and employees are always involved, whether
they are building a positive, liberating culture or a dysfunctional, fearful one. Certain steps must be taken if you want to
be engaged in developing a strong, sturdy culture that maintains
equilibrium, agility, and reliability.

The first step to construct a healthy culture is trust. You must
have it to give it away. You must trust to be trusted. You either
have trust or fear. Trust that by adjusting your internal belief,
you will be able to ask for what you want with confidence and
have a greater chance of receiving it. We don't need to fix the
outside world to feel safe. It's an impossible task anyway. What
we actually create is a scarier world by dealing with the people
in a nondirective or overpowering way. We can repair our inside
world, and then it won't matter what is happening in the outside
world. As we face and move beyond our fear, there is always
some level of stress.

Saving the first dance for you means caring for yourself while
you care for others. Maintaining a healthy mind, body, and spirit
is key if you're going to be there for others. After you understand
the way to be firm within and flexible with the outside world,
you know how to maintain your frame of reference. With that
awareness, we will move to the next chapter to learn the steps to
make your dreams a reality.

Questions to Explore

1. What motivates you or gives you energy? Examples might include exercise, meditation, nature, people, deadlines, your values, caffeine, status, or adrenaline.

2. What are your personal and/or professional strengths?

3. What activities would you like to be doing if you had the time?

4. What prevents you from doing the things you love to do?

5. What motivates you to keep doing the things that fill your day?

To receive your free gift worth $29 go to
http://www.SavetheFirstDanceforYou.com/relaxation.htm

IV.

Learn the Steps

When you dance, your purpose is not to get to a certain place on the floor. It's to enjoy each step along the way.
Wayne Dyer (1940-)

Finally, my instructor said as he demonstrated, "Let's start with foxtrot. Maintain your dance frame and move your right leg back so your toe touches the floor first. One slow step back, then move your left leg so that your toe taps the floor next to your right foot and to the left foot quickly and move your right foot to the left quickly. Move the left foot forward slowly with heel touching first. Move your right leg so your toe taps your left foot quickly, then right foot follows quickly. This forms the box step. Repeat this pattern—slow, quick, quick, and slow, quick, quick. Move your right leg back—slow, quick, quick. Then forward—slow, quick, quick."

It was as if my mind and body were totally disconnected. I was awkward. My dance frame and balance were hard to maintain at first. I felt a little embarrassed walking around the dance floor with my arms out at right angles. My thought went to the image of my instructors who moved with such grace and beauty. I continued as I focused on the possibility of what could be. I was sure that, with time, what I saw in those mirrored walls would become a prettier sight.

My instructor interrupted my intense concentration. "Keep your eyes up. Do another basic step now by continuing backward slow, slow, quick, quick, starting with your right leg. Turn around the room backward."

My brain froze with my body as I tried to listen and change the momentum from the imaginary box I was creating on the floor. I had to transform the imprint on my brain. In slow-motion, I started moving back—slow, slow, quick, quick. Would I ever get this? Would it ever become second nature? I used to think I was a good dancer. What happened to that? Now I could barely walk, much less dance.

My thoughts and attention were broken again with, "Move forward—slow, slow, quick, quick." As the evening continued, I could hear the music in the background, but I made no attempt to match what my feet were doing with it. I wondered when I could add this seemingly very important part of dancing to all the rest that absorbed my mind.

Only when the patterns become second nature are we ready to dance with a partner. There is just no way to bypass hard work. You hold your arm above your waist and move around the floor, consciously creating the patterns over and over. You rotate with your knees bent and your upper body lifted up as you move through the steps. With practice, it becomes effortless.

Because these dance patterns are wonderfully transferable, you can use them for many different dance rhythms—the waltz, rumba, or tango—and it all begins to make sense.

In the next phase, you dance with different partners to help learn the steps and to practice following and giving leads. Without all this practice, dancers stumble over each other. This isn't much fun to watch and it certainly isn't fun to do, but it is necessary. In a studio, the newer dancers stumble a little or repeat the few familiar patterns over and over. Practice, practice, practice.

How would your life be
if you set goals, took action, created new possibilities by
knowing what you wanted, and stayed focused?

As nurses, we have a general goal to help our patients get well and move beyond the need for our care. We have an unwritten goal to successfully get through the day, but what about our personal and long-term goals? When we want to achieve something for ourselves, starting with a written goal gives us clarity and focus.

One nurse had a goal of getting her degree. She had young children and didn't know how she could fit her goal into her schedule. She wrote the goal down, looked at the reality of her situation, and explored options for getting her degree. She was working two days a week in the middle of the day to cover for the lunch and dinner hours. As she explored the situation further, she realized that with the approval of her manager, she could take classes in the morning and arrive at work in time to cover lunches. Because she had taken some classes before becoming a mother, she was able to finish her degree and enter into a management position when her children went to school.

Another nurse wanted to spend more time playing the organ. She did some investigation and got a job at a church. Not only was she able to play the organ, something she loved, but she also was paid to do it. She became great friends with the choir and kept her nursing job as well. She would often sit in amazement when she realized that once she wrote the goal, looked at the reality of her situation, saw the options she could pursue, and identified what she was willing to do, she was able to make a plan that fit her lifestyle amazingly well.

There are specific steps to take when you're ready to create something new for yourself and your life. It is worth taking the time to learn them to bring your dreams to fruition.

Nursing Dance: **Knowing the Steps**

As in dancing, there are patterns in the nursing process: assessment, diagnosis, planning, implementation, and evaluation. These steps always have the same pattern, starting with assessment. A complete assessment involves a review and physical examination of all body systems plus an evaluation of the cognitive, psychosocial, emotional, cultural, and spiritual components of the individual. Next, the nursing diagnosis is the identification of the type and cause of the health condition, using clinical judgment and critical thinking. The planning phase involves establishing the priorities of care, writing goals, selecting and converting the nursing interventions into nursing orders, and communicating the plan of care. During the implementation phase, the plan is put into action to promote the desired outcome. And finally, in the evaluation, the extent to which the established outcome has been achieved is determined.

You spend years in school learning and practicing these steps. You have instructors and nursing veterans who inspire and encourage you to execute the steps with independence and ease. You repeat the same steps with every individual and gain confidence; you start with a dream.

Nursing Dance: **Start with a Dream**

Before your first dance lesson or nursing class, something important must happen. A dancer or nurse must have a persistent dream of seeing herself or himself as a dancer or nurse. Much hard work and practice is necessary to accomplish your dream, so you must begin with a full commitment. What keeps you going is your mind's picture of success. Imagination is a powerful dream maker. Vision comes from within. Hard work makes dreams reality. Positive thinking keeps you going through difficult times. Belief in the dream sustains you. You will feel resentful fulfilling someone else's dream for you unless it becomes your dream for yourself.

Identifying your dream is an important step. In *Captivating,* authors John and Stasi Eldredge describe the desires of a woman's heart. A woman wants to be romanced, to be part of an adventure, and to bring beauty into the world. Since nursing attracts mostly women, these are three areas to explore to determine what your dreams contain. In the work environment, romance would not exist in a conventional way. We would convert this desire to something that is more practical. Nurses want to be sought out for counsel. They spend all day with the patient and want to be asked their opinion and insight. If this doesn't happen or if their perspective is discounted or, worse, ridiculed, as the nurse your heart is in pain. If in her home life she is not respected, asked for counsel, and not romanced, she is suffering often in silence.

Nursing can be a great adventure of identifying maladies and guiding people to wholeness. You want to feel like an integral part of this adventure and essential to the triumph of the exploration. If a nurse feels or is treated as insignificant, her heart is wounded. She is interested in the medical diagnosis as well as the nursing diagnosis. Too often the medical community doesn't even recognize nursing as more than a handmaiden's role. This perception is extremely piercing to the nurse's heart since she knows that her role is integral to the successful outcome of her patient's hospital stay and healing.

The nurse's desire to bring beauty into the world is in the form of making the world a better place—one patient/person at a time. She wants to create a calm, safe environment for her patients to heal. If she can't construct this because there is tension or conflict, she is extremely distressed, even if it is totally out of her control. She is on a quest to generate what she knows is vital for the restoration of health and feels like a failure if she can't establish it.

Often nurses who are hurting leave the profession. The therapeutic environment becomes unsatisfactory to them. Often, their home lives are complicated, and their ability to keep giving without being refilled is prevented.

Nursing Dance: **Heal Your Heart**

The major problem nurses face is the need to heal their hearts. But their external focus prevents them from knowing the anguish inside them. It is so easy for a nurse to see the needs of others, and it pains her to not fulfill them. She has dedicated her whole life to this end. Gratifying people's needs is her duty. She can't allow people to suffer if something can be done and she can do it. She is surrounded by needs both at home and at work. Even though this eventually will deplete her reserve, she will continue to give until she is giving from her fabric, her very essence. When this happens, she is beyond exhaustion and withdraws in an attempt to stop the bleeding of her energy that is needed for her very survival.

Something needs to intercept this process in a proactive attempt to create inner harmony and a feeling of success. Knowing that the answers lie within and having a guide to create personal victory provide a place to start. Then you can make your dream a reality.

Nursing Dance: **Make Your Dream a Reality**

When you're ready to make a dream come true, start by setting a goal. A goal is the statement of what you want to achieve. As David Campbell says in his book with the same title, "If you don't know where you're going, you'll probably end up somewhere else." Research done at Yale on goal-setting found that only 3 percent of people write specific goals. Predictably, these are the most successful people.

I recently attended a recruitment and retention conference that provided a great educational experience. But how many people implement what is taught at conferences? We always feel so motivated, and then we get back to the real world and quickly become caught in inertia and blocks in the system. To grow and improve takes an internal motivation, and setting goals makes possibilities become actualities.

Creating a plan is something that must be given time and space. The process of actually completing our goals is even more demanding, and yet it can be done if the actions are studied and pursued. The first step to healing our profession is healing individually. We begin by asking ourselves what we want. This is the blueprint for our quest. There are specific things to understand if your intention is to grow. GROW stands for goal, reality, option, and will.

Nursing Dance: **GROW**

You may have heard of the term SMART goal. A goal that is Specific, Measurable, Attainable, Relevant, and Time Specific is most likely to be realized. How we make a goal measurable is by giving it substance. "I want to earn more money" doesn't have as much substance as "I want to earn $45,000 per year" has. Next, ask yourself if you can attain that goal. If you were setting a goal to go into nursing, it would be realistic. You must also determine if the goal is relevant or meaningful to you. If you don't care how much you earn, you won't be willing to make the necessary sacrifices to achieve your dream. Time specific is the last issue to address. If you want to earn $45,000 within five years, you have time to investigate and go to school. Your SMART goal becomes, "I will earn $45,000 per year as a nurse by January 20. . ."

To make a plan to achieve your goal, you must assess your present situation. I have a sailor friend who said. "If you think you're in New York and you're really in Virginia, you will never reach a target across the Atlantic. You'll be off by hundreds of miles even if you do all the other calculations right." This is true with everything you want to accomplish. Take time to face reality about your situation and any obstacles that you can foresee.

Next, look at your options and ask yourself what you would do if you knew you couldn't fail. Stretch and free yourself to list every possibility at this point. Then determine what you're willing to do to achieve your goal. Planning for the known obstacles will allow you to build solutions. Then look at the personal benefits of achieving your dream. Remember that WIIFM—What's In It For Me?—is always in effect. We don't do anything that doesn't give us what we want. We can't get excited about something if we can't see the benefit.

As the final step, think about who will support and encourage you to hold yourself accountable to the necessary tasks while you work toward your goal.

Nursing Dance: Choosing a Supporter

Whether in your role as a caregiver or for your personal goals, find people who will be your supporters or mentors. Know your values and don't ask support from people whose values aren't consistent values with yours.

Someone of the same sex who is willing to develop a deep relationship is preferable. It isn't good to develop this kind of close relationship with people of the opposite sex unless it is your spouse or perspective spouse because it can be misleading. People who are primarily interested in what is advantageous for them would not be good choices. You want to find a nonjudgmental person to help you accomplish your "to do" list. Don't be open with people who are willing to point out the splinter in your eye when they have a log in their own. Some people aren't careful about trampling on things that are important to you. Take the time to know what you want and then find just the right person to support you.

Of course, there are different levels of openness in relationships. Social relationships have very little depth. Some friendships have enough depth to share thoughts and feelings. However, the type of supportive person I'm suggesting can see the best in you and encourage you without judging. I'm describing a mutually authentic relationship in your inner circle.

Ask yourself if you have any authentic relationships that allow for total openness without fear. Some people are indiscriminately open with everyone, only to find that insensitive people are constantly hurting them. Be prudent about the level of your openness. Remember, you cannot have an authentic relationship if one person wants to look good and the other person wants to be authentic. It is lopsided and won't work.

A Nurse's Story

The first time I was in an authentic relationship, I realized how freeing it was. I accomplished so much more when I wasn't worried what the other person thought. In the past, I would choose goals or tasks that I really wasn't committed to. Oh, I would get them done, but feel resentful because no one appreciated what I did. Even worse was the feeling I had of being bad. I was constantly doing things for other people so I could feel good about myself. I realized that when I spent time and searched my heart for what I really desired, I got it done without needing other people's approval. For the first time I wasn't performing because it was right or expected or needed. I was doing what I felt drawn to do and it made all the difference in the world. I began to feel happy and got real joy out of just getting out of bed each day. My life grew easier and more manageable. I wish I had understood this years ago, but I just didn't see what I was doing. If I didn't have someone in my corner when I felt so challenged and frustrated, I wouldn't have been able to make this transformation.

When we are stretching to be transformed, we need to have support.

Nursing Dance: Know How to Support Your Goal

Maybe your goal is related to your marital status, relationships, child rearing, prayer life, work life, education, fear of conflict, anger problem, or other challenge. Ask yourself if you need simply a peer to support you in that area or if you need to find a coach who can walk you through the whole process. Or, do you already know someone you respect and could draw from in this particular area?

Consider building new relationships or moving an existing relationship to a new level. Take the time to imagine the individual who will provide the needs you've identified. Search for opportunities to develop peer relationships with those around you.

A Nurse's Story

I was looking for someone to develop a peer relationship with and as I was contemplating, I got a letter from an old friend I hadn't talked to in a while. When I called her, I began envisioning our working together. When approached, she agreed. I supported her and she supported me. It was a wonderful partnership.

Specific relationship-building exercises can be used when starting with a possible peer mentor. Make sure you have fun while you see if there's chemistry between you. Explore moving your relationship to a deeper level. Start by sharing a positive major event in your life. Just relax and enjoy the process. You can do this in person or over the phone.

Since creating new possibilities takes lots of energy, having someone in your corner is a big advantage. Maximum growth is not achievable alone because we all need support and encouragement.

Connect with someone who can help you stay in touch with what you want to accomplish. Accountability is critical to accomplishing your goal as is taking responsibility for your thoughts, feelings, and actions. It would be worthwhile to reflect on what accountability means to you. Actually, accountability is not nagging or being controlled, shamed, peer pressured, exposed, or even feeling guilty. If you have had toxic relationships with a parent, teacher, or coach, you may have such negative thoughts.

Healthy accountability is the desire and willingness to report our progress to someone we value and trust. This should not be given lightly to just anyone. This form of accountability creates an atmosphere for growth, safety, and empowerment. Our old relationships with accountablity against our will or from authority figures is not included here. If there is judgment in accountability, you create a harsh relationship. If it is too forgiving, the goal may not be accomplished. This is why choice is so important. Remember that choice must be made freely and fully to be successful. Accountability can then bring safety, empowering and energizing us to create. A healthy peer relationship challenges us to transform without punishment. Ultimately, if we are going to achieve anything in life, we must take responsibility for our own results.

Nursing Dance: **Know Who Is Responsible**

Your support person is not responsible for answers or making sure things go right. Since our belief about the capabilities of others directly impacts their performance, you want to choose someone who holds you in high regard and vice versa. In a peer support relationship, the goal is to build up each other's self-belief, acting as a mirror. It has nothing to do with controlling each other. For people to build their own self-belief, they need to know that their success is due to their own effort. Ownership comes from choice.

Don't suppose that you need to know the answers for someone else. Sometimes when you think you've judged the situation correctly, you might be projecting, seeing your own issues or your own positive and negative traits in another person. At times we displace our patterns of feelings and behaviors originally experienced with significant figures from childhood. The old saying, "I'll believe it when I see it" really is "Believe it and you'll see it." Become aware of your practice of projection and resolve instead to believe in yourself and your ability to heal and reach happiness beyond your wildest imagination. Believe in the people you serve and you will be helping them more than you can envision. We all need sustenance and alliances while we work toward our aspirations.

A Nurse's Story

I was having difficulty with my husband, and asked a respected person to support and encourage me through the process. My first thought was to make sure that I was giving my husband enough compliments a technique I had heard would help. When I began to explore this idea with my peer supporter who had resolved issues with her husband, I uncovered my real doubts. I didn't see how compliments had helped in the past. I would become resentful when I gave them because my husband didn't give them back. I felt responsible for his level of well-being. After our peer discussion, I realized I needed to work on me. I began a routine of getting up every morning, reading from a meditation book, and having quiet meditation time. I decided to let my husband take responsibility for his feelings. Amazingly, my relationship with him improved anyway. When things weren't good, I had developed a way to feel OK with myself, even when he was unhappy with me. Since I had been so focused on fixing our relationship, I wasn't taking care of myself. While I focused on the positive that had nothing to do with anyone else, I increased my self-esteem and realized that I had no control over his reaction to me. It had a wonderful, calming effect on me, which helped me feel better about everything else in my life. It's amazing how detaching can help you reconnect in a genuine way.

A Nurse's Story

I started exercising and my knees began to bother me so much that I didn't think I would be able to continue. When I talked to my peer, an experienced exerciser, she asked me if I was stretching. Interestingly, the next time I went to the gym, I ran into a trainer who gave me a half hour of free advice on how to stretch and get the most out of my exercise routine. I was soon exercising three times a week and able to work around my schedule. It's funny how hard that used to seem. Now, I just wouldn't know what I would do without it. The one critical question from my peer changed everything.

Creating something new takes focus, determination, and a person in our corner cheering us on.

Nursing Dance: **Stay Focused on Results**

You can do anything if you stay focused. Having someone for moral support and encouragement makes a big difference. We all need encouragement, especially when times get tough and we need to persevere. It's even better if our supporter has done it before us and knows the pitfalls. If you want to be a nurturing parent, find someone you admire as a nurturing parent to mentor you. Ask if the person would be willing to hold you accountable and share his or her steps to success. If he or she is available and willing—great. If not, keep looking.

Maybe you need to set a goal to find a mentor to help you get a new promotion. This person doesn't have to be in nursing, but it helps. Start by identifying what you need to do, such as taking some classes to learn necessary skills for that position. Then ask your supporter to hold you accountable.

Sometimes a person in a leadership position you desire will mentor you. This is different than a peer who supports, encourages, and holds you accountable for things you have identified. This kind of mentor is usually more directive and instructive, which can be more helpful in some situations. This form of mentoring is wonderful, yet today it seems to be a lost art form. Nursing needs this form of mentoring and there are attempts at making formal programs. However, the relationship building is not always extensive enough.

In some cases when we are supporting someone, we are functioning as a coach, much as we are our patients' coach. According to *Coaching for Performance*, certain important qualities are essential in a coach: patience, detachment, supportiveness, interest, perception, awareness, self-awareness, attentiveness, retentiveness, and the ability to listen.

When acting in this role, realize that problems can only be resolved at the level below which they manifest themselves. Notice things and provide feedback to the person. Ask how things are going. Ask for his or her perspective. Ask the person to reflect on related problems or patterns he or she sees.

Coaching is founded on asking people what they want and think rather than telling them what to do. Using these same concepts can help you coach your patients to achieve their goals for wellness. While you complete your nursing process, you need to involve your patients in every step.

Help them define their goals and break those goals into manageable chunks. Help them understand their own expectations.

Our short hospital stays today are actually beneficial in returning people to their daily routines. Discharge needs to be planned for from the beginning. Let's face it; people don't function as well in the hospital. With long stays, they may become confused and lose hope. Believing in your patient's ability to heal is one of the foundational steps to healing. Being supportive, encouraging, and helping them understand the concept of how expectation, accountability, and authentic relationships will aid their healing process.

Nursing Dance: Know Your Expectations

Expectations influence our thoughts, feelings, behaviors, and attitudes. And whether intentional or not, attitudes can significantly impact others. Some expectations are unspoken and need to be uncovered. Unrecognized expectations can foster negative attitudes.

When we clearly define and communicate expectations, we are more likely to have a positive attitude and enjoy greater satisfaction even if the expectation is unmet. Help your patient and peers identify their expectations.

While you learn to use these powerful concepts for your own personal growth, you will be able to pass on the steps to others. When you teach something, it reinforces what you know.

What happens when we achieve our goal? We may actually experience a period of mourning. Our goal has died by becoming a reality. This subtle emotion may go unnoticed or come as a complete shock. We expect to be happy when we achieve a long-awaited goal. Our support system becomes extremely helpful in this process.

The key is being able to honor and share our feelings. After the recognition and acceptance of where you are has occurred, the way to move past the mourning phases of grief is to take another dream off the shelf and create another goal. As we continue the cycle of striving to expand and grow to our full potential, life emerges as a great adventure. And we never have to stop growing.

Nursing Dance: **Never Stop Growing**

You will always need the skill to take your dreams and make them reality. For example, the initial goal of earning $45,000 per year will only motivate us through nursing school and earning a reasonable income.

In fact, the biggest challenges arise after school. You find yourself with fragmented knowledge about diseases, the nursing process, and medications. You know how to do many tasks, but not necessarily how to put them all together.

To feel comfortable with skills you must encounter many situations, because every patient has specific needs. You will always have challenging tasks or relationships at work or at home for which you will need support and perspective. All challenges can be overcome with vision and a support system.

You have the foundation from your education to accomplish tasks. You're part of a team and a system. Nursing is about relationships with other nurses, healthcare providers, families, and patients. You need to give and receive support from the system. Trust is built in the relationships with your patients and coworkers by following through, spending time pondering what needs to be done, asking for what you want, and accepting that you can't always get everything you want.

Be committed to continuous new possibilities. Change is the only constant in the world today. Creating something new takes tremendous energy, and most of the energy is used while you're identifying what dream you want to make a reality.

Nursing Dance:
It's Like Going Up a Steep Hill at First

You will eventually get to the top and plateau, so you need a regular source of refueling. It takes about six weeks of rigorous effort to shape a new behavior. The energy required to maintain it may be less, but some of us have tendencies that will need our focused attention forever. Ask yourself what rejuvenates you, make a list, and refer to it often.

In this chapter, we discussed the steps for dancing, nursing, and achieving our hearts' desires. Remember, we perform a dance within us that takes precedence over the dance with others. Just as the dancer needs to practice the steps alone, we need to practice before we can do the steps with others, walking before we dance. Intentionally walking our walk and dancing our dance alone allows us to be more fully present and authentic when we're with others.

The steps to achievement allow us to have fulfilled dreams. Remember, we can't give what we don't have and we can't teach what we don't know. The steps to accomplishment for our patients lead them to healing and wholeness. Common ground is where we meet. We always follow the patient's lead.

Nursing Dance: **We Follow the Patient's Lead**

We get on board in the direction the individual wants to go. We need to be grounded, balanced, and know our own soul position. We get support from the right kind of people as we open ourselves to transformation. We guide others as they create their goals. We act as coaches who build up or break down, depending on our focus and actions.

Successful people experience transformation and teach others to do the same. Confident people know when to lead and when to follow. The next chapter we will discuss how to know whose leading and who's following.

Questions to Explore

1. If you could do anything with unlimited resources, what would it be?

2. What makes your dream so meaningful, fulfilling, or exciting to you?

3. What does your spouse, peer, coach, or friend think about it?

4. What do you need that you don't have to move forward?

5. What has prevented you from doing it in the past?

To receive your free gift worth $29 go to
http://www.SavetheFirstDanceforYou.com/relaxation.htm

V.
Know Who's Leading and who's Following

The dance is a poem of which each movement is a word.
Mata Hari (1876-1917)

My instructor walked up, put his right hand on the middle of my back, and took my right hand with his right. We were moving through the same dance patterns together.

"The woman is the star of the dance," he explained. "The gentleman guides her through the dance steps. The woman gives her partner resistance so he can direct her. Opposition allows each partner to know the position of the other. The gentle pressure allows steering to transpire. The man has to be steady, agile, and alert to keep the dance exciting. The woman must be stable, nimble, and responsive to cues. Dancing is two autonomous beings coming together as one. Their union activates the dance. Each dance is unique due to their blended gifts."

I was lifted off the floor. My body tingled. He held me in his arms and we moved across the dance floor with a smooth gracefulness I had only imagined. It was exhilarating. Alone, I was mechanical and focused on steps and patterns. Together, the beauty of the dance was expressed and experienced.

All my practice suddenly made sense. I knew why one partner's instability could produce disaster. We were two fully centered individuals who were totally present to each other. We were aware of each other and ourselves at the same time. It felt effortless, until suddenly I lost track of what I was doing and we hit a bump in the dance floor, so to speak.

At that point, my self-talk took over. "What is wrong with me? I am never going to get this. I don't pay attention. When am I going to get this right? If I don't stop this, I'm never going to be a good dancer." I wanted more of the feeling of oneness, so I reconnected and went back to work with my steps and patterns.

Ballroom dancing takes time and discipline to learn. The leader and follower have mirrored steps. The leader walks forward while the follower walks backward and vice versa. The follower is dependent on the leader to channel her through obstacles. The follower and leader both must be confident in their individual steps. At times the lead will pivot as the follower walks around. The leader needs to be the forerunner and prompter. The follower needs to distinguish the lead and counter.

The dancers must work together as a team. Each of them has to practice independently for massive lengths of time. Needless to say, individual rehearsal is not the most pleasurable ingredient of instruction, but it is necessary. The unification is enhanced and more striking than either is in isolation.

How would your life be
if you knew that leaders allow themselves to be transformed
and by doing so give others permission to be transformed?

In the hospital, many situations present themselves. Sometimes we lead; other times, we follow. We have a choice to be a leader and be proactive or to follow the other person's lead from a position of strength. Most difficult situations can be extinguished through our creative response.

One nurse worked on a chronic pain program for several years and did most of the orientation for her unit. She felt frustrated because there was so much to teach and she had so many other responsibilities, including taking care of patients. She began to systematically write down the things she did on a typical day each day of the week. Then she wrote down the exceptions and within a month she had a comprehensive orientation manual. She found nurses referred to the manual when rotating to her unit or when performing unfamiliar tasks. Instead of being the unit people avoided, there was a waiting list of willing staff. She reduced the time of new employee orientation by half. Realizing she loved teaching, she took a formal education position and created a procedural manual and a process for developing and supporting nurse educators.

A physician yelled at an ICU nurse for calling him with patient issues. Many of her coworkers avoided calling him as much as possible, which often put their patients at risk. One day she listened quietly as the physician yelled. After some time went by, he asked if she was still on the line. She stated, "I am writing what you said to me in the chart." She never had a problem with the physician again.

Let's put dance into nursing terms. The nurse is the star of the hospital. The physician guides the nurse through her steps by ordering diagnostic tests and medications. They are two autonomous practitioners with complementary bodies of knowledge. Giving adequate resistance presents itself in the form of perspective.

Nursing Dance:
Get to Know Each Other's Viewpoint

Knowing each other's viewpoint allows you to respond to ever-changing patient needs. The nurse spends the most time with the infirm, so his or her outlook is essential to the physician's plan of care. High-quality patient consideration is realized by working together. Before the nurse is able to respond to situations with clarity, she must know herself and what drives her. We continue to re-create reality according to what we have learned to expect. We lead the dance unconsciously.

Nurses are nurturing and compassionate by nature. However, nurses frequently have come from harsh circumstances that lead to compulsively doing and caring for others as a way to create a safer environment. I am not saying that all nurses come from abusive or extremely dysfunctional situations. However, many do. The human condition sets us up for the triangle of distress.

Nursing Dance: Know the Triangle

Ordinary maturation results in all people being wounded. Viktor Frankl, who survived the Nazi concentration camps, observed that abuse victims answer this insult with either care giving or abusiveness. Just as in the case of widely publicized sexual abuse, some turn out to be victims, while others are converted into predators.

What frequently transpires is a relationship triangle in which each individual revolves through the roles of victim, rescuer, and prosecutor. Both the victim and the rescuer resent their role and ultimately become prosecutors, exhibiting either overt or passive aggression. The cycle continues without conscious awareness. Each easily recognizes the role the other is playing and is unaware of or justifies his or her own. Leading and following rotates from partner to partner.

A Nurse's Story

My husband was much better at computers than I was. When something went wrong with the computer, I became helpless and couldn't think clearly. When I asked for his help, he would complain that I was interrupting something important and responded resentfully. If he couldn't fix it quickly, I would get angry. Of course, this made him less interested in helping me the next time. I soon realized that my anger began just at the thought of asking for help. Underneath the anger, I was afraid that he would not want to help me. This interaction happened over and over. Since I never got help from my parents, I harbored resentment that I unconsciously was unleashing on my husband. Actually, I was acting like a victim until he would rescue me and I became the prosecutor. Now, after my increased understanding, I can ask for help without being a victim.

Her husband's side went like this:

"I would frequently be angry at my wife if she needed help with her computer. It always seemed to happen at the worst time. When I helped her, she never seemed to appreciate that I was in the middle of something else. I felt bad about getting angry and yelling at her. Because I couldn't think clearly when I was angry, it took longer to fix the problem, which made me even angrier. Becoming aware that the underlying cause of my anger was about my parents ignoring my interest, I recognized that I was taking that out on my wife. I was playing the role of the rescuer and became the prosecutor when my wife needed help."

As described, both the victim and the rescuer have an underlying rage that has nothing to do with the situation. Their rage affects all situations until it is healed. While we cap it as much as possible, we carry out our drama with someone with a mirroring wound, which doesn't solve the problem because they are not the source of our pain. Healing is an inside job and requires taking responsibility for your own feelings and discovering their origin. Remember, when you point your finger at someone else, three point back at you.

Projecting our issues on others solves nothing. If you find yourself blaming others for your feelings, you miss the opportunity to learn about yourself and heal.

A Nurse's Story

I was getting angry at people for not appreciating what I did for them. I realized I was really angry at myself for doing things I didn't want to do. I thought I was angry with people for asking. I lived in a cycle of being either guilty or angry all the time. Finally, I dealt with what drove me. At the root, I was afraid of people's rejection, so I wouldn't do what I wanted. Though hard and scary, I faced my fears and became freed from constant turmoil. Now I don't need anyone to stop asking. I just need to say no when I want to. I can't tell you how it's changed my life.

Many nurses lacked nurturing as children. Instead, they often nurtured their parents and siblings. Many had alcoholic, neglectful, and/or abusive parents, only to marry similar partners. Amid the dysfunction, their mothers may have spent all their energy just keeping the household going. The child was expected to help carry the heavy burden. The ones who had the natural gifts of compassion and being of assistance were rewarded in some way. The nurturing child instinctively understood that he or she was seen as good only when care giving. Helping became synonymous with good. Not helping was equated with bad. Doing for himself or herself was associated with bad. To offset the guilt about being bad, they cared for others.

This pattern can occur totally unconsciously. The individuals aren't aware that when they do something for themselves, they feel selfish. Any hint that someone else thinks they are selfish will stimulate an underlying rage that may be covered up with more doing. Yet these people are either unaware of their anger or they turn the anger inward if they believe they are not doing enough for others.

The reason they get upset when people take advantage of their kindness is unidentified. They are not mindful of their external need for appreciation to make up for the lack of internal approval. Unhealed people want outsiders to be pleased about what they do because they may resent doing it or don't appreciate themselves. It's time to break out of these old patterns.

Nursing Dance: Breaking the Old Pattern

Patterns can only be broken by facing the reality of a situation. If you take time for yourself and feel guilty or bad, you compulsively become more giving to stay ahead of the feelings of badness. You can't see this vicious cycle. The only way out is to stop and let the feelings catch up. But the fear of being bad is so great that slowing down is not considered an option.

Over givers usually find over takers to share life. The two can flip back and forth in these roles. The one who plays the over taker is only too happy to give the over giver grief if he or she is not doing something for the over taker. So, every time the over giver does anything that is not caring for the other, the over giver is told about it in subtle ways.

One person might have a massage. The partner complains about the money spent. Another person takes time to play golf. The partner complains that the family is lacking due to the absence. This situation produces fear of authenticity, causing denial or hiding. This describes the plight of the workaholic. The addiction is too excessive working in order to avoid feelings or thoughts of badness. Eventually, the cover blows up anyway because no matter what you do, someone can always find something to complain about. Heal the wounds and no one will have the ability to induce guilt that results in compulsive behavior.

Start by facing two facts. Thoughts and feelings are transient and you own them. That doesn't make them universally right, so other people don't have to agree with them. The people or outside sources are not the cause, but do stimulate our feelings in the present moment. Our reaction is due to a pattern set earlier. If you run from or try to eliminate your thoughts and feelings, you become addicted to whatever you used to avoid them.

Addictions take many forms, including drugs, alcohol, and work, eating, and gambling. Some more subtle forms such as people addictions and doing good works for others can be just as difficult to break and much more difficult to see.

The substances or activities make us feel better about ourselves.

For over giving, we are rewarded by the outside world. Why would your family want to tell you that you are doing too much for them, even if they recognized it? They stand to lose all your good works. For the compulsive do-gooder, the activity has been so long standing that it seems natural. These people may start sensing frustration, resentment, or anger and not see that they are creating the situation by not facing their fear of rejection. Constantly feeling bad about themselves when they are not doing something for others, they do more to feel better.

The cycle is created: doing, becoming angry for lack of appreciation, getting away from that person, feeling guilty and going back to repeat the cycle again. They keep stretching themselves to do more than they really want to do. However, like a rubber band, you can only stretch yourself so far before you snap.

Maybe the snap happens in the form of emotional breakdown, depression, or physical pain or illness. The unconscious drive is to take care of oneself. I was one of these people.

I was working full time as director of surgical services, working on my master's degree, was married, had a ten-year-old son, and was playing the role of Superwoman by volunteering at church and my son's school. I had dinner on the table every night, went to soccer games, cleaned my own house, wrote my papers early Saturday mornings, and took classes every other

Friday night and Saturday while my son visited his father. I was efficient.

It wasn't until I finished school that I collapsed. I didn't want to do anything. I had to take a month off from work after having some difficulty with my new boss. I didn't want to clean my house, make dinner, or see friends. I was exhausted. Things started falling apart, but I had no idea what was happening to me. I didn't know that the healthy part of me was screaming for me to slow down and take life easier.

My response was to change my environment. I got a different job within the hospital and pressed forward. I didn't take the time to figure out what was really going on within me. It took years to see my internal process. I was so aware of what other people needed. It pained me not to help, so I kept doing, resenting, withdrawing, and feeling guilty.

I still have to resist the temptation to respond in the same way, but at least I own the process now. I acknowledge that it is my way of interacting with the world. My anger is my signal that I don't want to do what I am about to do. Choosing to honor my feelings and understand how they work for me instead of against me is freeing. Instead of hating myself for getting angry, I view my anger as my indicator to stop and think about what I really want to do. I no longer blame others for taking advantage of me because I know they can't without my permission. I am not compelled to do what I'm asked. It is my choice. Understanding ourselves as the cause of what happens in our lives gives unlimited power through choice.

Nursing Dance: **Recognize the Underlying Cause**

As nurses, we replay our childhood neglect, abuse, or invasion in our intimate relationships. If our home lives are not extremely supportive, this area may often drain us. Since we are so used to doing everything, we choose partners who depend on our strength. Some of us are even the primary breadwinners while we still play a major role in the care of the family. As one nurse said, "I work hard all day taking care of others and then I go home and continue working hard, taking care of my family. There is no time for me."

With so much to do, there is no time for anything that doesn't include taking care of others. This arrangement seems rewarding as long as we think it is perfectly all right. Only when we sense a personal unmet need do things begin to fall apart. We often don't develop support systems to take care of ourselves because we never acknowledge the need. We believe we have always taken care of ourselves. But actually, we buried our needs underneath our self-sufficiency. If we were invaded as children, we never made our own decisions, and we followed our parents' guidance. We were fine with this system because this is how they showed us love. We might not uncover a problem until death takes them away from us and we feel lost. For the first time, we recognize that we don't know what we want except to please them.

If we were neglected or abused, we took care of ourselves. We never depend on anyone and everyone can depend on us. All is well until the defenses we created start crumbling. For one nurse, it was the death of her parent. For another, it was her kids leaving home. Another got ill. Still another had a difficult situation at work.

Whatever triggers the collapse can be overcome by facing the truth. There is a plan for each of us. Hold this truth as your foundation, have a heart that wants the right thing to be done, access wisdom, and have faith because it allows you to move mountains. Four forms of faith need to be acknowledged as you move beyond your self-imposed boundaries.

These are the faiths we taught the patients in our chronic pain program: faith in your plan and process of transformation, faith in the people you bring into your life who help you, faith in your own ability to heal and transform, and faith in God to be your pathfinder. Taking the step to venture into your unknown is easier when you know the process for becoming an authentic person. It requires openness to yourself and your support system. If you find unsupportive people surrounding you, develop or find a new circle of real friends who are honest, loving, and open.

Nursing Dance: Be Open to Love

Having more love and intimacy in our personal lives allows us to be more resilient at work. Feeling loved is so glorious that we fear losing it. We can continue to unintentionally re-create situations in which we don't feel love in hopes of feeling love this time.

Unfortunately, our history may block us from receiving the love even when it is offered, and our unconscious resentment of the past keeps the cycle going. So when we receive love, we can't accept it or are afraid it won't last. We don't know how to become intimate with others because we're missing some lower needs of trust and safety.

Opening ourselves to love that is ours for the asking can fill the void. Just as we block it, we can unblock it. The key is available if we learn to turn it. This condition will affect our home and work life. When we are overworked on both fronts, we are sure to head for breakdown, which may come in many forms.

We have all experienced working with the walking dead. They come to work everyday, negative, unengaged, and difficult to ignore. Yet that is what we try to do. These people have no safe haven, so they stay disconnected and believe they are right about all their negativity.

Improving your personal life will benefit your work life. In his book *Love and Survival*, Dean Ornish explains that we can become more intimate with our loved ones by sharing our wants and feelings. Most of us are fearful because sharing what we want makes us vulnerable. The other person has the ability to say "no" and we will consciously feel the pain of not getting what we want.

Many of us have heard that sharing our feelings can improve our communication with our spouse. However, as Ornish explains, we often share our thoughts disguised as feelings. We say, "I feel you shouldn't open my mail." Or, "I feel that you made me afraid." These are thoughts camouflaged as feelings. They would likely be heard as judgmental or fault-finding. Sharing a feeling would sound like "I feel invaded and angry when you open my mail." Or, "I feel afraid and want to get away from you when you are yelling." The first examples gave away responsibility for feelings; the second maintained ownership of the feelings. It's essential to face our true feelings head on.

Nursing Dance: Face the Truth

Another area to contemplate is accepting divergent feelings. People feel totally differently about situations. We may not even realize this because we may surround ourselves with people who agree with us. We may be so blind that when someone gives us another opinion, we think the person is purposely taking a different position to irritate or undermine us. A particular situation does not produce predictable universal feelings, even when we get to know the person well.

We need to recognize that we don't cause other people's feelings; we trigger them. When we have an unhealed issue, we will continue to bump into it until we resolve the underlying cause. Two improvements in our relationships are possible for our unhealed issues. We can become conscious and be open to transform what negatively affects the people we love, or they can heal and no longer be affected by our actions. This, of course, works both ways.

Do you see yourself being victimized? A major issue that blocks our fun when working or living with others is being the victim. When you play the victim, you always need a rescuer. Both the rescuer and the victim will eventually become the prosecutor. Victims resent their rescuers and rescuers resent their victims, so they prosecute each other by pointing fingers at the flaws and place blame. Getting out of the cycle demands focusing on what you're contributing instead of on what the other person is or is not doing to you.

I became conscious of how I created this dynamic with my husband while working on a big project. I was feeling stuck and afraid that my results were not going to be good enough. I talked to my husband and decided to pick him up from work, rather than have him take the bus. On this Friday evening, he suggested that we do something together. He was in a "let's get the weekend started" space and I was in an "I'm scared to death about next week" space. After I picked him up, I began to complain that he wasn't appreciative enough of what I offered. He became defensive because it would have been OK with him if I hadn't offered it. We found ourselves in gridlock. I was sure he was insensitive and ungrateful. He was confused and hurt. The closeness left and each of us was sure it was the other's fault.

The next morning, I kept wondering what part I was playing. I became aware that I was playing the victim instead of saying what I really wanted, which was to continue working on my project. I could have asked him to come home on the bus and make dinner when he arrived. Instead, as I played the martyr, I judged him as taking advantage. In the past he had been happy to do what I asked. In this instance, I didn't get what I wanted because I didn't ask. Even more, I made things worse by blaming him for being insensitive. I can't tell you how hard this was to admit to myself, much less to him. When I finally got the nerve to share and take responsibility, we were both freed from the oppressive feeling we were experiencing.

This kind of interaction can happen in our professional life too. There is so much to be done and the needs of people never seem to stop. If we are not honest with ourselves about how much we want to do, we become victims and blame our state on others. Learning what really works will set you free.

Nursing Dance: **Learn What Works**

Although it is necessary to address your past, it is not worthwhile to keep replaying how and who wounded you in childhood. You just become a victim. Self-help groups where everyone sits around bemoaning victimhood are useless. It is only worthwhile to recognize your story and move on to what you're going to do about it. Whenever you're overwhelmed with feelings, ask yourself what they are telling you and formulate a plan to address them. Make sure the plan is something within your control.

If your answer is about how you're going to fix someone else, do not go there. If you think other people are being insensitive or inconsiderate, you're probably right, but what are you going to do about that? There are only three options. You can alter, avoid, or accept. Share your thoughts in a non-demanding way, and maybe those involved will be sensitive to your concerns. Or, break away from them and you won't be exposed to their behavior. Or, stay around, knowing their behavior may not change. Healing starts by recognizing the origin of your feelings deep within you.

A Nurse's Story

I got in touch with a feeling of wanting my mother in my crib and her not coming. I was overwhelmed with sadness and rage. I suddenly realized why I didn't expect to get what I wanted. I didn't get what I wanted even as an infant, so I stopped asking. I stopped wanting. I panicked at the thought of having a need because I would have to feel the deep longing for something that never came.

Whatever your story is, own it and honor it without judgment. Set yourself free by refusing self-pity. Sharing your story can be very healing if it is done for the purpose of moving beyond it rather than complaining. Because our stories are sacred, they should only be shared in a safe, loving, compassionate environment where great wisdom is available. My wish for you is to become the source of that secure, loving, compassionate environment where your own internal wisdom will prevail. Give yourself space to do so.

Nursing Dance: Give Yourself Space

Give yourself space where you can go to enjoy some quiet peaceful time alone. Separate from the hustle-bustle of the world regularly. We need time in nature to reclaim our soul and to identify our soul position. What do you know about your soul or your own uniqueness? That you are a completely distinctive human being? Do you appreciate that you are unlike anyone else on the planet?

Your whole being is irreplaceable because no one else has ever been like or will ever be like you. Take time out of your hectic schedule, commune in nature, and find out what you're going to do with your gifts while you're here. Think about the imprint you're going to make on the world that is inimitably yours.

You have access to everything you need. Healing starts with acceptance. Accept the love that is available to you. Feeling love from the source of all love, I have found, will set you free from a cycle of fear. You must slow down to feel it.

Accept that you are not bad; you are wounded. Every child has been wounded in some way. Uncover the gift by accepting that painful feelings offer an opportunity to heal and move beyond them. You may have been working on making the outside world safer for yourself. Instead, use the outside world as your resource and source of knowledge. It has information that you need. Stop and read the vital signs of progress.

Nursing Dance: **Take Your Pulse**

Stop taking everyone else's pulse and take your own. Take time every day for quiet to sense wisdom from within, from the source of all wisdom.

You create your own sense of safety. No one can fashion it for you. When you become more loving toward yourself, you will generate surroundings that reflect that. When you demonstrate more compassion concerning your strengths and weaknesses, you will see how both operate for you. The result is your own secure reality.

When you know yourself, you are able to respond to any situation that may arise. You are able to take action appropriately without overreacting to other people's behavior. For example, when someone is being hurtful and undermining others, the whole nursing staff needs to stand united against it. Don't let one person stand alone. If one of the old guard puts all the new nurses through the wringer, let that person know it is unacceptable. Don't look away and say, "Oh, that's how Jean is." Tell Jean she is running off the new nurses and she needs to be more supportive. Jean may not even be aware of what she's doing if you don't tell her. If she gets defensive and leaves, that is her concern and may be better for the department. Whatever you do, make sure your motivation is clear. Don't use your workplace as a place to complain and point fingers at everyone else. Put a stop to backbiting. Stop the constant complaining. Be open to new directions. Then you have time to work on the important things. Past behavior predicts future behavior unless you take a proactive approach to transformation.

Nursing Dance: **Behaviors Are Predictable**

You can work together to improve your work environment. You will be able to take better care of patients who desperately need your help. You are capable of seeing the benefit of perspective that differences bring and make your department unique. Take time to identify the behavioral styles that you bring to your venue. Certainly, some people will be easier for you to work with because certain behavioral styles are naturally easier than others. Yet all styles have important contributions and can work very effectively together when you understand the unique differences.

We behave very consistently in the way we communicate with others, both verbally and nonverbally. For instance, during a staff meeting, you may see four different styles. Some people will give only the bottom line and the big picture. Others will ask lots of questions. A number will change their mind about decisions. Some will speak only when asked. The healthcare work environment is complex and challenging.

To become more effective in communicating with others, become more aware of how you interact and relate. Generally, we interact in four basic ways, according to the DISC profile. These are known as dominance, influence, conscientiousness, and steadiness. These four behavioral styles combine in each person to create complex yet predictable behaviors. The goal is for all staff members to share freely from their unique perspectives. When you are able to empower individuals to contribute and feel valued, loyalty to your team is shaped.

An individual with a high dominance behavioral style places emphasis on shaping his or her environment by overcoming opposition to accomplish results. These individuals have a tendency to get immediate results, accept challenges, make quick decisions, and question the status quo. These folks desire an environment that includes power and authority, opportunities for individual accomplishments, and freedom from controls. They need people around them who weigh pros and cons, calculate risks, and use caution since they tend not to focus there.

Individuals with a high influence behavioral style place emphasis on shaping the environment by influencing or persuading others. Their tendencies include contacting people, being articulate, and creating motivating surroundings. The desires of these individuals in the workplace would include popularity, social recognition, freedom of expression, and group activities outside of work. They need others around them who concentrate on the tasks, speak directly, and respect sincerity.

Those with a high steadiness behavioral style usually place emphasis on cooperating with others to carry out tasks. They have tendencies that include performing in a consistent, predictable manner, demonstrating patience, and developing specialized skills. These people desire an environment that includes maintenance of the status quo unless given reasons for change, predictable routines, and credit for work accomplished. These people need others around them who react quickly to unexpected change, stretch toward the challenges of accepted tasks, become involved in more than one thing at a time, and apply pressure on others.

Characteristic of a high conscientiousness behavioral style places emphasis on working conscientiously within existing circumstances to ensure quality and accuracy. Their tendencies include adhering to key directives and standards, concentrating on key details, thinking analytically, and weighing pros and cons. They desire an environment that includes clearly defined performance expectations, values of quality and accuracy, and a reserved, businesslike atmosphere. These individuals need others around them who delegate important tasks, make quick decisions, and use policies only as guidelines.

You can become more effective by identifying your behavior style and what naturally enhances your performance. You can discover your own style by completing a profile at <u>www. SaveTheFirstDanceForYou.com</u>.

The next important step is to work toward consciously achieving enhanced performance. Everyone can become more aware and effective with increased personal knowledge and development. The number one controllable nursing issue is our perception of a relationship.

Next, it is vital to concede that the other person's perspective is not bad, it is just different. When we transform, it is amazing how different the world around us looks. Understanding your behavioral style improves relationships at home as well as work, thus allowing you to generate relationships that are gratifying.

Following the lead of a physician doesn't make you a handmaiden. You each have autonomous roles. Someone must lead while someone follows. The patient is the ultimate star. The healthcare professionals guide them through the dance. You have to know your own moves. You must teach them their steps to better health. In this way, you lead through serving others.

Nursing Dance: Be a Servant Leader

You are a servant leader with the goal to lead your patients to improve their state of health. You lead for the sole purpose of helping others. You must know your patients' present health status and understanding with the intention to guide them in the most beneficial direction. You must focus on how receptive they are and what kind of support and encouragement they need to move forward.

It is important to know your role in every relationship you have within the hospital. You are the patient's advocate. Never lose focus of your significance. This is the source of your confidence. Appreciate the joint values and goals you share with your colleagues in helping the people who have entrusted their well-being to you and work together to enhance the health of your patients. Your missions are linked. Your patients will benefit.

You are a leader, whether you are giving a medication or providing much-needed patient education. Leading and following are part of the dance. Both are hard work and both are essential.

Quality of care requires an interdisciplinary methodology. Collaborative partnerships build trust. Always remember you must have trust to give it away. If you find that you have an issue with trust, work on it. Don't go searching for trustworthy people. Look within yourself and heal your trust issue. Celebrate progress with your patients and partners in health care. Continue to educate yourself, your patient, and the people around you. Take time to honor what you bring.

Nursing Dance: Honor Your Contribution

A Nurse's Story

I realized one day that physicians have no idea what nurses do. They think we are here to carry out their orders. I wanted to change that kind of thinking, so I asked if we could do some nursing research on the care of urinary catheters. It was approved and we were able to reduce the number of urinary tract infection in catheterized patients.

Necessity is the mother of invention. When you want to do something positive with a frustration, let it serve a purpose. Don't get mad; get constructive. Get involved in nursing research. Show why nursing is important and help your patients. Eliminate activities that don't work. Discover ways to enhance outcomes. Openly communicate, keep your attitude in check, listen intentionally, and be responsive to your patients and those around you. You can assume this approach if you have truly taken care of yourself and saved the first dance for you.

After understanding the intimate link between leading and following, you are ready to connect with your partner.

Questions to Explore

1. What kinds of people and/or situations frustrate and produce stress for you?

2. How long have you been feeling this stress?

3. If you didn't have stress, how would your life be?

4. How will your life change when you reduce your stress?

5. What would your life be like if you didn't get rid of your stress?

VI.

Connect With Your Partner

**If you cannot get rid of the family skeleton,
you may as well make it dance.**
George Bernard Shaw (1856-1950)

My dance instructor greeted me at the door. "Welcome to your first studio dance. You will have many partners tonight, and I want you to remember two things–keep smiling and keep moving."

We made two circles, men on the outside and women on the inside. The men were directed to move to the right and, when the music changed, to dance with the person in front of them. My first partner was bearing down on me so hard I felt man-handled. The next was so spongy that I had no idea where we were going or what I was supposed to do.

This man was followed by someone who confidently directed me around the dance floor. I knew exactly what he was trying to lead me through until I missed his lead. I was a little befuddled, but I kept my smile and my feet moving. I looked like I was doing some kind of pretzel dance as my body with my two left feet moved in ways I was sure was not anything like ballroom dancing. I just kept moving, smiling, and laughing at myself. Yes, I was embarrassed, but what could I do? When the music stopped, I apologized and waited for my next partner. Our sweaty palms met and we were off. It all but overwhelmed me, but I was certainly more motivated for my next lesson. Then my instructor became my partner and things got better. I was comfortable with the steps he led me through. Wow, what a relief.

Had I forgotten everything I learned when I couldn't follow some of the leads? The different kind of energy of each partner affected me tremendously. We had an energy exchange. Sometimes I felt afraid, other times frustrated, sometimes uplifted, and at times embarrassed. I apologized when I missed a lead. I would smile even when I knew I received a bad lead.

We were all novices, learning to dance with different people, and needed encouragement. We could choose to refresh and boost each other with our positive regard. We fashioned the dance based on our ability to interact with each other. Only hard work would eventually make the dance look effortless.

The process of connecting with my partner in a meaningful way seemed to take so long but when I did, it felt fantastic. The continual exchange of energy flowing while we performed the dance made me feel alive and animated. My partner's responsiveness was exciting, the harmony between us strengthening, and the movement of our bodies with the music invigorating. The sense of being mirror images motivated me to stay focused and connected. The experience elevated me to a higher level.

Practicing with a partner made it even better. A well-rehearsed dance team was transforming. As the anxiety of my uncertainties dissolved, I could focus on our mutual goal and just have fun. I felt like I was floating. It was electrifying.

Doing a variety of dances with different kinds of music was thrilling. When the music changes, you stand for a moment, allowing yourselves to feel the music, get in your dance position, and begin. Many of the steps are transferable from one dance to another. The mixture of music and dance keeps things stimulating.

How would your life be
if you learned about yourself through relationships
and recognized that the way you feel about others
tells you about who you are?

When you are authentic about whom you are you're able to share your needs and expectations in a non-defensive and effective manner. As a nurse, you deserve to be treated with respect and courtesy. When people don't do that, it is helpful to have support to walk through fear and ask for what you want.

And then expect the best.

A nurse who frequently worked with new nurses felt compelled to inform them about their flaws, their need for more knowledge, areas needing improvement, and how things were "supposed" to be done. In other words, she had the reputation for eating her young. New nurses were frequently in tears after spending time with her. Not surprising, the department had retention issues and a high turnover rate. One gutsy young nurse decided to take responsibility for creating something new. She asked the other staff members to back her up when she asked for different treatment, and they agreed. Within a month, she became personal friends with the "nurse of doom and gloom" and things began to change. Together they identified the best instruction practice to support and encourage while holding new nurses accountable. The transformed nurse soon became an advocate for new nurses. Turnover rates dropped and the complete nursing staff became part of the retention solution.

Another nurse went to a healing touch seminar. She asked a patient if she was willing to experience one of the techniques. The physician came into the room while the session was going on and the patient explained what was happening. The unhappy physician went to administration to report the nurse for performing a treatment without a doctor's order. Recognizing that healing touch was a new technique, the nurse knew there was more education to be done. When the physician told her she was to "follow doctor's orders," she asked the nurse executive if she could start a committee of physicians, nurses, and other healthcare providers to research, evaluate, and regulate complementary/alternative therapies. The committee wrote up a protocol describing how caregivers and patients would receive, be informed, or request such therapies. As a result, the therapies became a formal part of patient care along with a brochure that described them.

We experience an energy exchange with everyone in our lives. In nursing, some patients drain your energy and others uplift you. Our home life also has a great impact. If you're struggling with old issues, your spouse, children, or lack thereof, you also may sense a level of strain in the workplace. You must understand your internal condition because it impacts your relationships. Keep moving, smiling, and even apologizing if it's hard to follow the lead.

Nursing Dance: **Teamwork**

Be totally honest with yourself. Own what you are bringing to the situation and continually work at clearing your blocks and healing your wounds. Honor wherever you are. Listen to your feelings and respect the great insight they have to give you. Be authentic. If you stay diligent and strive to understand all the ways to work well with others, you will enjoy the benefits of having a collaborative workplace. With practice, you will make it look effortless.

In the workplace as in dancing, teamwork is essential. Donald Egolf has written about four predictable stages in team building: forming, storming, norming, and performing.

Nursing Dance: Forming

In the first stage, the team is forming. Members are getting to know each other. They begin to recognize and value each other's contribution and expertise. The team members must learn to trust and depend on each other. They need to understand what they can and cannot expect from one another. In such an atmosphere of support and encouragement, everyone thrives.

Nursing Dance: Storming

Next, the team goes through an inevitable stage of storming. This stage is unpleasant emotionally and many members of the team try to avoid it. A natural response to the diversity in the team is some level of conflict. Defining roles and reconciling philosophical disparities is critical. If the team has a clear objective and is able to find common ground, people move through this phase quickly. Failure to take time to honor everyone's needs and to openly deal with conflict will result in dysfunction of the team. Facing sensitivities and differences openly will allow the team to move beyond this phase quickly and effectively.

Nursing Dance: Norming

If the team is able to move through the stages of forming and storming, the third stage of norming will be in reach. At this point, team members know their work schedules and routines to follow. Guidelines with written expectations should be available. The team is aware of each other's roles and responsibilities. Differences are transparent and accepted. Optimally, open discussion has been established as a norm for the group to air further differences. People feel comfortable with each other and are ready to get the job done.

Nursing Dance: **Performing**

Once the team has successfully progressed through the first three stages, the group is ready for performing. The team becomes productive and able to achieve goals easily. Making changes as needed and processing through obstacles that may arise in everyday activities are negotiated without difficulty. When all is well, the team feels cohesive, bonded, and successful. If a new member arrives, the team will regress to an earlier stage, but usually the stages will not take as long to advance.

Nursing Dance:
Understand Your Team's Approach

During the performing stage, each individual's natural approach and preferred role on a team become evident. Some have a conceptual approach, enjoying the discovery of ideas. When presented with a new situation or problem, they like to investigate options and talk about ideas. They can imagine the master strategy to overcome obstacles and are focused on the future and solutions.

Others have a spontaneous approach, wanting freedom from constraints. They tend to move from one subject to another and work on multiple things at once. These people can be impatient and don't feel a need to follow conventional thinking. They are guided to decisions by their feelings.

Still others take a normative approach. They like the familiar and rely on their past experience in similar situations to guide them. Accepted norms and expectations direct them. They like to know the consequences of their decisions before they act and let others take the lead. These folks seek to fit in with others.

Finally, there are people who have a methodical approach, preferring order and rational thinking. A step-by-step process where they can examine options and think things through serves those best. They are careful and focus on what they can support with proof. To see things fit together in an orderly way is very satisfying to them.

All of these approaches come together in a way that is very beneficial to an organized team. When your department has an issue, it is wonderful to know what people do well so you can empower the members to achieve the best results. Those people who have a combination of conceptual and spontaneous approaches are the creators. They are the ones you want to look at the problem first. They will reframe the problem and look for solutions that are unusual and unique. Fresh and original is what you can expect from people in this group because they are unrestrained by fear of failure and boundaries. Because they like ideas, this group may move through many thoughts without stopping and eventually lose sight of the real objective.

Once great ideas are offered, the next group, known as advancers, continues the process. Being spontaneous and normative, these individuals add their insightful ability to plan. Using past experiences and successful methods, they offer excellent guidance. Although they prefer familiar ideas, they don't let boundaries discourage them. This group will direct their thinking to achieve objectives in the most straightforward and efficient way. They also help others see the possibilities and help carry it forward. If left alone without others with a strong conceptual approach, the advancers could implement concepts that are not completely thought out.

Further in the process, refiners look at the problems and suggested solutions to evaluate the consequences and prepare for surprises. This group is methodical and conceptual. You will find them comfortable playing the devil's advocate to test soundness of ideas. They will challenge the concepts and analyze the information in a logical way to spot any potential failings. Good at reviewing viewpoints and plans, they will modify and create new ones to ensure successful execution. If allowed to control the group or the process, the refiner may lead the team toward choosing low-risk ideas, filtering out ideas that may have greater risks but better payoffs.

Next, the executors follow up on team objectives and realize solutions. They strive for achieving enhanced outcomes with a concentration on the detail. The executor prefers to let others take the lead, enjoying the task and responsibility of final implementation. People in this group may have little interest in the group discussion. They prefer proven, familiar ideas over novel and untried ones. This group is methodical and normative. Cautious and careful in their approach, they will think things over before proceeding and implementing something that is not workable for the group. Left without other approaches, they may lose sight of the goal and pursue irrelevant strategies.

When these patterns combine into one that is adaptable to all approaches, this is accomplished by the flexors. This group will monitor the contribution of the other team members and contribute wherever needed to keep the process going in the right direction. Able to fluidly move from conceptual, spontaneous, normative, and methodical approaches, they are essential to the overall productivity of the team as they play three or four roles during the team processing. They understand the perspectives of all the team members. Unless a well-defined role in the team is assumed, others who are more strongly committed to their own role of creating, advancing, refining, or executing may ignore the flexor. To be able to identify your role in solving problems and resolving situations in the workplace, you may wish to take a team assessment at www.SaveTheFirstDanceForYou.com.

Embracing each nurse's approach to a given situation improves the team's ability to work together while conflict becomes accepted as a natural part of the process.

Nursing Dance: **Conflict Is Inevitable**

Conflict, like the finger-pointing that occurs from one shift to another, is inevitable on a nursing unit. It can be constructive if its source is understood and responded to effectively before it spirals and becomes overwhelming. If not, it can be a major hurdle that will prevent the team from successfully performing. One nursing director had an open forum for complaints and issues. She had a page for staff to write concerns as suggestions for meeting topics. It produced tension at first, but soon open, honest sharing began to occur. She also asked each staff member to read and sign a commitment to coworkers to provide excellent care and strong teamwork adapted from Marie Manthey, author of *The Practice of Primary Nursing.*

Conflict can arise from many sources. Author Mary Ann Anderson points out in *Nursing Leadership, Management and Profession Practice for the LPN/LVN* that some people are incompatible. Members of the family may not even remember what the dispute is about, but all their lives they have been involved in interpersonal warfare. They make a choice to be contrary. This is also evident in sex, race, or age discrimination situations. Another example might involve two people in competition for the same position. Obviously, handling these situations in a direct, caring way is essential.

Sometimes work groups struggle with the distribution of scarce resources. If one group gets a raise that is inconsistent with other groups, conflict is provoked. Getting specific days off during the holidays can produce extreme tension among the staff. People may join the workforce having had scarcity in childhood and interact in the work setting with a mentality of scarcity.

Any time people have opposing needs, drives, wishes, or demands, whether they are internal or external, the possibility of disagreements exists. Helping people work through these issues allows the team to refocus on the important matters.

Hostile encounters are another source of conflict. If two people apply for a job and one aggressively tells the other that he or she shouldn't apply for the position because of lack of background and/or the skills necessary to do it, the results can be explosive. A person can be passive-aggressive and talk about another to anyone who will listen. Individuals might even go to the person making the hiring decision and tell him or her about a lack of competency. Because both aggressive and passive-aggressive behavior is damaging to individuals and organizations, it must be addressed as quickly as possible.

Role confusion between RNs and LPNs on a nursing unit can also cause conflict. If an LPN occasionally substitutes for an RN, a strong potential for an unclear role exists for the LPN. The best way to manage this is to give clear expectations about what part of the role will be covered during the assignment. Unmanaged situations of this sort can result in power struggles. Frank communication can demonstrate to the individuals involved that their skills and abilities are acknowledged and appreciated.

Sometimes, individual needs for togetherness and aloneness can result in conflict. Some people like to go to lunch alone and prefer working with clients independently instead of the team approach used by the rest of the staff. These people may not participate in staff meetings or join group parties. They may be distant from others. This can result in other employees feeling left out or discriminated against. It's impossible to know the reasons without asking whether the person who does not act as part of the team feels insecure or overconfident. Further, negative feelings from the rest of the staff must be addressed to reduce clashes. This effort is time consuming yet necessary.

On the other hand, some people want to be too close at work. Although initially this may seem positive and caring, when people think their coworkers are family, it is problematic. The activities and conversations of the work team should remain professional. Personal comments can undermine the way people think and the level of confidence among team members.

It takes time to determine and be receptive to how people think and feel. Educating individuals about the dynamics and the conflict that may arise is challenging yet rewarding, and essential for healthy teamwork.

Sometimes, people have a sense that an argument is happening between team members even though nothing has been observed. Other times, people believe others are upset with them. This perceived or sensed conflict can destabilize the effectiveness of the team. Having one-to-one conversations with the individuals involved can help deflate the tension.

Unresolved conflict is destructive to any work setting. It can result if someone is aggressive and devaluing to another person and the devalued person doesn't have the skill for conflict management or doesn't want to be involved in a dispute. This happens in the nurse-physician relationship because the physician frequently has more clout in the hospital. The nurse holds in her feelings, and attempts to bury them. Trying to manage unsolved feelings about being treated aggressively by another person takes a lot of energy. The person is constantly playing a tape in his or her head about what should have been said or could have been said. This kind of behavior can go back and forth until people wear out, move on, or give up and see themselves as losers.

Nursing Dance: Effective Partnerships

If you want to be part of an effective partnership, whether it is in a dance studio or healthcare setting, you never want to be hard on yourself or your partner. Connecting with a partner takes a high level of consciousness, intense work, and sensitivity. We all have days when we feel grumpy and are tempted to take out we negative attitude on others. But if it becomes a habit, eventually no one will want to dance or work with you. It's always important to apologize and to take care of your grumpiness some other way.

Often, familiarity breeds contempt. We feel we have the right to take out our bad feelings on the people close to us. Husbands and wives who decide to take dance lessons can be pretty horrible to each other. These couples will never become great dancers if they don't get over it and show respect and sensitivity toward each other. Likewise, if people at work conduct themselves in conflict-producing ways, they will never be part of a successful partnership.

Time is necessary to know the feel of your partner. You have to understand the appropriate lead for each of the steps and know how to respond appropriately and quickly. This interaction happens fluidly and effortlessly when you have been practicing with your partner for a long time.

First, you need to recognize what you are doing that benefits or hinders the relationship. With confidence, you can easily transform a poor lead into a first-class result. Watching movements of a more advanced dancer helps you visualize your desired result and then feel it within yourself. We communicate with each other through our resistance. Resistance is a normal natural part of the dance if we don't make anyone wrong for their resistance.

Nursing Dance: **Communication of Resistance**

The resistance that each partner holds against the other allows the synchronized movement. If one partner does not hold his or her dance frame or resistance, the balance is knocked off and dancers are ineffective. The tension within each partner and the resistance between partners allow them to be aware and focused. If pressure stops or is inconsistent, the trust between the partners is broken and the dance is hindered.

As a nurse, you have many partners. In an inpatient setting, you partner with your patients as they try to learn how to return to wholeness. You partner with other staff members on your unit to accomplish all the tasks of patient care. You partner with the pharmacy to get the patient's medication. You partner with physical therapy, radiology, laboratory, transportation, other nursing units, and physicians, just to name a few.

Each partner has a different style that requires you to respond appropriately for best results. If you are trying to be what people want instead of being you in all situations, you will be giving inconsistent pressure, which has the same negative effect on the partnership in the hospital as it does on the dance floor. It is essential to know yourself and honor who you are as you relate to others.

In dance, one person always leads and one person follows. The same thing is true for nursing. You need to know when to lead and when to follow. As in dance, the leader has to know the steps and be thinking about the next ones to offer the proper lead. The follower doesn't necessarily have an easier job; the leader experienced the same process, but from the opposite perspective, knowing what was coming and responding accordingly.

In nursing, you have to know the steps to care for your patient. You need to complete the activity at hand and prepare the next step in the plan of care. You need to be sensitive enough to your patient's lead that you can respond appropriately. You must keep moving because you can't accomplish the goal if you don't. If you keep smiling, you will find more enjoyment in your coworkers and the process. In one study, people were asked to put a pencil in their teeth so that it created a forced smile. Others were asked to put a pencil between their lips so a frown was created. Both groups were instructed to watch a video. The group with the forced smile consistently enjoyed the video more than the group with the frown. If you want to enjoy your life more, start by putting a smile on your face.

When you acknowledge what you like about your partner, you are more likely to improve the connections. If there is something you want, ask for it in a positive way. Be sensitive and make a request in a way that doesn't criticize but is encouraging. Think about what you want to accomplish, not about what is wrong.

When you want to communicate, make sure you have a positive connection. Begin by thinking about what you like about the person. Making reference to what you can achieve together will bring the person closer to you. Think about how you feel when someone has good things to tell you versus when someone has a list of things you need to fix or of things you don't do well. You want to get away from the person with the negative list and spend time with the person who has good things to say.

If you communicate when your partner is not in a good place to listen, you will simply waste your time and energy. Doing this long enough will exhaust you. You may find that it just gets harder and harder to communicate because your partner is resistant. Just as the amount of dance resistance is important, too much resistance will make other partnerships off-balance and ineffective.

Sending out energy without real purpose will drain you and make you unwilling to try again. You will lose confidence. You will feel unsuccessful and decide that it is no use to undertake anything else.

Your partner won't know where you are if you don't have a consistent pattern of communication. Reliability builds trust. This is why it is important to do some individual practice communicating before you try to communicate with someone else.

Visualize the free exchange of ideas without making someone wrong for his or her perspective.

Nursing Dance: See Your Success

See yourself being successful. Many of us imagine how the other person is going to get upset and by the time we say something colored by our underlying fear, the other person does in fact get upset.

Imagery is powerful. Research has supported this. One group of athletes mentally practiced successfully making basketball shots. Members of another group went to the courts and practiced their shots. When the results were compared, the groups were equally successful at making basketball shots. What we imagine, we create. Recall that after I watched a professional dance showcase, I imagined myself being like the dancers and before long I was able to move in very natural ways.

Our internal communication begins with pictures. We visualize ourselves doing what we want to accomplish. Sometimes fear paints that picture as a negative outcome and we create that conclusion. Fear brings past hurts and resides in the future. When we live in the future with fear, we create repeated negative results. It is only when we face our fear, challenge our fear, and overcome our fear that we can make different choices and generate what we really want.

Ask three close friends to visualize the perfect workplace and to describe it. Each person will visualize something differently because of his or her own perspectives. Communication has two important components known as sender and receiver. The sender needs to take the time to know what he or she wants to say by visualizing it and creating a receptive environment. When we communicate, we each get our own picture based on our own perspective. Make sure the people with whom are talking understand what you mean so you both hav same picture. Many miscommunications are just the result of the receiver getting a different picture than the sending was trying to convey. Presenting clear thoughts is essential so that your partner understands the meaning.

Believe you can have what you want, state your request clearly, and make sure the receiver understands your request. People filter what they hear through their belief system. You only have control over your belief system; you do have some influence by holding the receiver in high regard. Receivers will color your message with their thoughts and feelings. If they sense safety with you and your desire for their higher good, they are more likely to listen, even if the message is not something they want to hear.

People usually prefer specific guidelines or information rather than vague, undefined expectations. If you want to improve performance in another person, it's important to share your desires in a positive light with the belief that you will get the results that you want. Otherwise, you may feel disappointed in the poor job the receiver did by your standards, while the person believes he or she did a great job by his or her own standards.

Think about your intention before you speak. Know what you want to accomplish before you formulate the words and take action. As always, save the first dance for you.

Connecting with a partner requires focus on knowing yourself, appreciating your partner's contribution, and acknowledging your common goal. To build a team that is based on trust and intent on achieving success, you must understand your approach, role, and communication style. Once you are connected to your partner, you are ready to hear the music.

Questions to Explore

1. What relationship would you like to improve?

2. How are you in that relationship (defensive, aggressive, a victim, hurt)?

3. What do you want the relationship to look like?

4. What have you done to make your relationship wish come true?

5. What would it be like if you were still here or still in this situation in five years?

To receive your free gift worth $29 go to
http://www.SavetheFirstDanceforYou.com/relaxation.htm

VII.

Hear the Music

Who hears music feels his solitude peopled at once.
Robert Browning (1812-1889)

Holding our positions, we waited to hear the music. Our waists lifted and chests proud, heads tilted slightly to the left, belly buttons to spines, knees flexed, and our bodies connected at our diaphragms. My husband extended his left leg and I matched the move with my right. Within moments, we heard the three-quarter-time of the waltz. As the music filled us, we took pleasure in the view below from the top floor of the Bank of America building.

Ooonee…two…three… Ooonee…two…three. Our knees released slightly, giving us an upward movement on the ooonee… as we traveled confidently around the smooth dance-floor. We journeyed effortlessly in perfect complement to each other and the music with a room full of observing eyes on us. I felt enchanting. Our years of practice allowed us to experience this level of connection.

I was internally energized and externally moving with grace-ful ease. The preparation and attention to detail had all been worth it. I was transformed into an exquisite butterfly suspended above the world. The music shaped the dance and created some-thing beyond both of us. Its vitality guided us and our response created passion-in-motion.

How would your life be
if you recognized that the way you filtered information
creates your experience and you assumed that
whatever you believe you would see?

As nurses, it is easy for us to make assumptions about the motivations of others. We can find all kinds of evidence to prove our point about why a particular nurse or physician is mean-spirited. We each have a way of looking at the world that is supported by our facts. However, I encourage you to reach for something new. If you're not getting what you want, look for others who are and check out what they expect. We hear what we are listening for.

One nurse was known to yell back at physicians when she called them and they became upset. If the doctor said he would report her, she said she would report him. Her patients were usually very sick before she would notify the doctors. One of her colleagues suggested she just listen to what the physician had to say because the physician was helpful in giving instructions when she called him inappropriately. After some coaching, she realized she interpreted the physician's response through her filter "He thinks I'm stupid." She began to see that he and she just had different priorities. When she implemented her colleague's suggestion, she was astonished at the results. She actually became friends with the physician and found him to be a great source of information. Shortly thereafter, she was invited to be part of the hospital's physician relations committee and began going to other nursing units to describe the remarkable difference she found by listening instead of reacting. She felt proud to be part of the solution after having spent so much time being part of the problem.

Another nurse who didn't get her requested time off believed her new manager had a personal dislike for her. She spent time in the lounge talking about how she knew the denial was personal. Her peers had different perspectives, knowing there were many requests for the same time off. With some coaching, the nurse engaged her manager in a conversation about her unrealized request. Describing her struggle to give everyone their request and her first-come-first-served policy, the manager invited the nurse to create future schedules. This situation brought to light the nurse's childhood pattern of believing people didn't like her when her desires weren't met.

Recently, my husband and I took our six-year-old grand-daughter to the circus. I had forgotten how big a part the music played in the excitement. Dr. Phil says in *Self Matters*, "You either get it or you don't. Become one of those who get it." I watched my granddaughter move with the music. She gets it. Maybe it's because we've been dancing with her since she was a small baby or maybe she was just born with rhythm. Hearing music can be a learned skill. Even if you haven't been encouraged to move with the music, you can still develop rhythm.

Hearing music is paramount to dance and nursing. The ability to hear is the primary element of listening. We hear what we are listening for. Real listening is an active process that has the three basic components: hearing, understanding, and judging.

Nursing Dance: **Real Listening**

Our first goal as nurses is to hear what is being shared—to repeat the facts. You've heard the report on Mrs. Jones and you can reiterate the details. You've paid enough attention to catch what the nurse on the previous shift said.

Understanding, the next aspect of listening, happens when you interpret information. You hear that Mrs. Jones is refus-ing to have the tests that were ordered today. She has been a very receptive and compliant individual up until this point. You wonder why she refused the tests. You ask yourself if she is deteriorating.

Next, judging occurs. Did you believe what you heard in the report? You may have decided to check on Mrs. Jones as a result.

As a dancer, you must hear the music, understand what dance matches the music, and make a judgment to do a dance that matches the music. There is no beauty in dancing a foxtrot or cha-cha to a waltz. However, it is perfectly acceptable to choose among a cha-cha, swing, or foxtrot for some music. You may even decide to mix it up and do different dances during the same music.

To be in sync with the music and your partner, you must be able to hear the difference between the three-quarter-time of the waltz and the four-quarter-time of a foxtrot, or the difference between the roll of the tango and that of the cha-cha. As you're learning to dance, you're paying attention to the beat, tempo, and rhythm. You can do the same basic patterns of steps in different dances with subtle differences in the movement of your feet that construct the variations. In foxtrot, you tap your second foot against the first, while in the waltz you make a U-shape with your second foot, and in the rumba you move your second foot diagonally.

Getting started on the right beat takes time to learn. Dancers must be highly sensitive to the music. We interpret the music with our dance. Trusting each other becomes supremely important because either one of us can knock the other off the rhythm, affecting our ability to perform. All the requisites of the dance must be learned independently; their interdependence comes together with the start of the music.

Nurses have to dance to many different tunes. The tunes come from all kinds of directions and require changes in our responses.

Nursing Dance: **Know Your Filters**

We respond to people and situations according to our ability to hear through our own filter. Our capacity to understand is affected by our patterning. Our judgment to act is based on the message and our filtering patterns.

Albert Ellis developed rational emotive behavioral therapy. He describes three fundamental things that take place in response to any life situation. These are his ABCs. A stands for the activating event, an incident within our personal space. B is our belief or bias about that occurrence. C is the consequence, or our response to what has happened, based on the state of affairs and our belief about it.

We have no control over what happens to us. Our belief system or bias directly affects our response to the world. This is our filter. And this plays a big part in our response. The goal is to respond rather than react. When we respond, we give ourselves time to think things through. Reactions happen without thought and are complicated by unconscious past events.

It would be nice to think that we are totally objective, but it simply isn't true. It is estimated that people filter out or change the intended meaning of what is heard in 70 percent all communications. Remember the telephone game when we were kids, where one person started a message and passed it on to another and so on? The message was very different when the last person repeated it out loud.

Communication is a complex subject. Breakdown can occur in a number of places, including the sender, the sender's filter, the message, and the clarity of the message, the receiver, and the filter of the receiver. The sender must be clear about his or her message and aware of his or her filter when communicating and the receiver must know his or her filter and have the ability to interpret the message as intended.

Transforming our beliefs can result in many positive solutions.

A Nurse's Story

Several people before me had made mistakes that led to an error. The epidural was supposed to be hung in the post anesthesia care unit and I was flustered because I had never started a drip before. I asked for help, but no one was available. The pharmacy made a mistake by putting the wrong dosage in the bag and I was overwhelmed trying to execute the task. I didn't catch the medication error the first time I checked the bag before I hung it. When I rechecked the bag after starting it, I realized that the dosage in the bag was 1 mg/cc instead of the 0.1 mg/cc that were ordered. I was the only person reprimanded for the error since I was the last person who could have caught the mistake. I was devastated, although the patient suffered no negative effects.

When I first spoke with this nurse, she was filled with shame and self-hatred, even though the patient hadn't received even a fraction of a milligram of the medication when the error was identified.

In recounting the event, she stated, "I'm not a bad nurse." I responded, "You are not a bad nurse, and no matter what happens, this does not make you a bad nurse."

As she burst into tears, saying:

I was always blamed for everything that went wrong when I was growing up. Nothing I did was ever enough. I could never get anyone to see my perspective or give me the help I needed. I learned to take care of myself and do for other people. I felt awful most of the time unless I was helping someone and they were happy with me. I felt like it was happening all over again.

Times such as these can make or break a career. Making a mistake is devastating, even if no harm comes to a patient. When something like this happens, the music or self-talk that is your filter becomes very important to monitor. Filters guide your response. Childhood tapes saying, "You never get things right" or "You always screw things up," affect you for the rest of your life if you don't challenge them. Self-defeating beliefs may include thoughts that are constantly telling you that you're not good enough, you're not safe, or someone is trying to take advantage of you. Past failures and hurts create another filter that can cause a negative response to the world by saying things like, "We tried this before and it didn't work," or "Every time I try to talk to someone about something that bothers me, it blows up in my face."

You always have the option to turn a bad situation into an opportunity to grow. The nurse who made the medication error decided to share her story and heighten the awareness of other nurses rather than hide her head in shame. She began a medication error awareness program. She eventually became the safety officer and interfaced between the pharmacy and the nursing units, reducing medication errors throughout the hospital. Later, she received a patient safety award for her contribution to the hospital. She converted a negative circumstance into a positive result. She challenged her filter and consciously transformed. Once you have your own self-talk in check, you're able to remove your self-inflicted obstacles, and free yourself to work better with others. It's important to embrace your role and adjust as needed.

Nursing Dance: **Know Your Role**

Nurses, physicians, and other healthcare professionals have different scopes of care. The patient is best served when there is open professional communication among all caregivers. As a nurse, your most important role is that of a patient advocate. It takes a confident nurse to bring pertinent information to the physician's and other healthcare providers' attention. If you see yourself as the physician's handmaiden whose role is to carry out orders, the patient will not get the advocacy he or she deserves.

One nursing role that can become problematic is the compassionate nurse. Being compassionate is the wonderful gift of nursing, but it takes more. The gracious, compassionate nurse may take as many patients as given and never speak up about the safety issues that are involved with poor staffing practices. Some nurses say they leave an organization that has poor staffing rather than voice their opinion. This response is not being the patient's advocate.

The confident nurse knows when to step forward and make recommendations. He or she knows that working with colleagues is the way to get successful results. Taking time to brainstorm and solve problems is an important part of nursing. It is the only way to create solutions and guarantee future success.

Nurses are autonomous practitioners and oversee the care that is given to the patient. They are aware of the treatment plan and ensure the care is carried out. In this way nurses protect and save lives, fulfilling the role of watchdogs of the healthcare system. Inconsistencies and inadequacies must be identified and addressed or patients will suffer.

The confident nurse is not passive or aggressive. He or she is persuasive and persistent. If nurses are fearful or collapse when challenged, they will not be able to be the patient's advocate. One of the ways to overcome fear is to believe in your success before you achieve it. Many of us fear a bad result and then try to resist it. It is possible to strive for positive results and influence what actually happens. Nurses can set intention while they provide personalized care for each patient. Becoming aware of our beliefs allows us to adjust them as needed.

Nursing Dance: **Know Your Beliefs**

Knowing your belief system and maintaining a positive focus can have far-reaching effects. Your belief affects your patients. In my seminars, I have attendees identify the power of their thoughts. I have people get into sets of two and ask one of the duos to think of something positive. Then I have the positive thinker put out his or her arm and the partner tries to push it down. What people discover is they are strong when they are optimistic. The exercise is repeated with a negative thought and the muscles actually weaken. This exercise demonstrates that our thoughts truly affect our physical strength.

Interestingly, our thoughts influence others as well. Our belief about someone sets our intention. We can purposely do this and benefit our patients. Establishing a positive intention for your patients is about believing in their capacity to heal. You must believe that everything you do for your patient is for his or her higher good and increases his or her wholeness. As a nurse, you are licensed to touch. When you touch your patients, establish your intention for that touch to assist in their healing process. If you are not always holding your patients in the highest regard, you are working against them.

Intention is a very powerful part of nursing. Wayne Dyer speaks about living life with intention. Dyer, who spent his early life in foster homes, away from his mother and an absentee, alcoholic, often-imprisoned father, believes that we share an abundant divine force. He thinks that abundance in all things is possible for all of us. Take inventory of how you look at the world. Ask yourself if you give away your energy by giving up your optimistic stance. You have a choice to see the inequities and inconsistencies or abundance –for all. Setting intention is like making a wish and believing that it will come true.

Make a wish and believe in your own ability to heal your wounds. I have heard many nurses' stories. Many of them relate to their role as caregivers in childhood. Some parented their parents. Others were molested; some felt neglected and emotionally starved. Many did not feel cared for as a child or in their adult relationships. Everyone wants to be loved and understood. As a nurse, you give what you want to receive. When it doesn't come back, you bury anger and give more. You don't realize that you are reducing the chance of getting what you want.

We teach people how to treat us. When a child doesn't receive love, he or she feels unlovable. This makes an individual work harder and harder to be lovable in hopes of getting the desired love. But trying to be more loving and understanding with people who don't return it in a loving manner will exhaust all your resources. It doesn't work. We must do this in our jobs, but we often set this up in our personal lives as well.

Until you accept what is happening and make the needed transformation, you will not get what you want. The results will be resentment and fatigue. A healed person is naturally loving and accepting. He or she does not need to compromise to be loved and accepted. You may be compelled to be excessively loving and accepting, even when you don't feel it. This perspective motivates you to suppress feelings you see as negative or to strongly disapprove of yourself for having what you believe are negative feelings. In reality, all feelings are just expressions of you. If you find yourself judging your feelings, love that part of yourself. The more loving you are to yourself, the more naturally loving you can be to others.

People become bitter and resentful toward others who take advantage. Remember, no one can take advantage of us unless we allow it. There are no negative feelings. There are just feelings. There are only negative behaviors associated with feelings. Many of us resist feelings of anger. When we do so, we are really reacting to the negative behaviors we have seen associated with anger.

Separate feelings from behaviors. Embrace whatever feelings you have. Feelings are your source of knowing yourself, healing old wounds, and finding your path to consciousness. Take a look at anger to find areas in your life you have made wrong, are resisting, or with which you are uncomfortable.

Nursing Dance: Dealing with Anger

As you accept your feelings, you will eventually find your natural rhythm. Anger is one of the disturbances of the natural rhythms of our souls. It is a strident rhythm.

One Nurse's Story

I will never forget the day I really got in touch with my original source of anger. I had been consciously trying to find out why I was so unhappy when I had accomplished everything I ever wanted in my life. Something was missing from my life, and I realized it was me. I was so busy accomplishing tasks and taking care of everybody else that I didn't even know what I wanted for myself.

I had taken over my mother's role in childhood. I never did totally understand my mother, but I generally sensed I didn't get what I wanted from her. She and my dad fought frequently and then went on like nothing had happened. I took over the role of keeping my father happy so he wouldn't yell or hit everyone. Many years later after my dad died, I tried to tell my mom how much the fighting scared me and how alone I felt when no one ever talked about it. She basically told me to get over it since it was in the past. She said she loved my dad and didn't want to hear anyone say anything bad about him.

I was angry. I was scared. I was so sad. All these feelings were overwhelming, and I could feel the pain in my chest and diaphragm. My arms and legs felt like deadweight. As I sat with all these feelings without trying to justify why it all happened, I realized for the first time the toll it had all taken on me. I wasn't trying to understand or make sense of it. I just experienced the feelings.

A Nurse's Story

It occurred to me that I felt guilty for my good relationship with my dad because of the resentment my mom and sisters had toward me. I carried this into my adult life. I saw that I unconsciously made sure I was never too successful so that I couldn't move too far beyond my sisters. In subtle ways, I kept punishing myself for being in the enviable position I held in the family. I could see that I always seemed to undermine my success in some way and create some kind of unhappiness in my life. Something had to be going wrong in my life so that I didn't feel too much better off than the people around me. Of course, the cause of all this was unconscious, but I was conscious enough to see what I was doing way before I knew how to stop it. I spent most of my life feeling guilty. I felt angry at my mother and sisters for judging me.

A Nurse's Story

I had difficulty admitting anger for as long as I can remember. I disapproved of anger and I was deathly afraid of my own as well as others' anger. My father had violent anger. I really loved my dad and understood him very well, except for his anger. I was as if I completely disconnected from his angry side. I began to realize that this lack of acceptance and understanding created a response in me of complete collapse when I experienced a high degree of anger within myself. I felt guilty for being angry.

I thought anger was bad and if I felt it, I was bad. I was afraid that if I was extremely angry, I would repeat the expression of my father's anger. Whenever I was angry, I would just give up and get away from whatever made me feel angry. I tried to do everything right so no one would criticize me and make me angry. I suppressed my anger the best I could. I didn't realize until I totally faced the cause of my anger that I was everyone's puppet. Others could make me do almost anything just by yelling at me or acting angry toward me.

I was constantly trying to make everyone happy and I never did. My counselor was always telling me, "Don't give up. Give in." It was a wonderful freeing experience when I decided to give in instead of give up.

Giving in is acceptance while giving up is collapsing or denying our anger. We often want to stay away from our anger, but it is not possible to resolve our issues without facing them. Suppressed anger can be compared to the "beach ball effect." You can only push a beach ball under water for so long before it erupts. The further you push it down, the greater the force of the eruption when it comes up. Likewise, the longer you suppress anger, the more powerfully it will explode. The explosion will be in direct proportion to the amount of stuffing you have done.

Many nurses have had a lifetime of stuffed anger. Much of your anger is very legitimate. The problem arises when it is displaced onto other people and situations. You can tell this is happening when you see yourself overreacting to people and things around you. Some extreme cases result in violence in the workplace and road rage. It doesn't have to get this terrible to face your anger head on.

The book *Anger* by Leo Madow describes recognition as the first of four helpful steps in working through anger. You may need professional help to do this. Don't be afraid to seek it if you recognize these symptoms and can't get in touch with anger. Depression is often described as anger turned inward. It is also absence of feelings. Hospitals have employee assistance programs that may be a good place to start. Coaching can also uncover this block. Anger of which you are aware is much less harmful than unrecognized or un-admitted anger. It is essential to uncover your feelings to begin. Look for the words that express anger, such as disappointed, frustrated, let down, unhappy, fed up, annoyed, harassed, hurt, or ready to explode. If you feel guilty or sense that the anger is unjustified, you will pass judgment on your feelings and you will not be able to move past the first step.

Once you recognize you are angry, identify the source of the anger. This may be obvious or it may be very subtle. For example, if you are angry with your boss, you may displace your anger on coworkers, patients, family, or your children. You may feel guilty about anger toward your parents and find that you are aggressive toward older people. It may be difficult to acknowledge your anger especially if you think your parents had good intentions.

The source of anger may be obvious or seem to be obvious, but really may be displaced. Our spouse and children are often the easiest targets since they are close and give rise to our anger.

After recognition and identification, you want to understand why you are angry. Frequently, people overreact as a way of denying the opposite true feeling. The sweet person is not really sweet at all but a bitter, angry individual. Because we sense this contradiction, we find such people distasteful to be around. A mother can be overprotective to cover feelings of resentment toward a child. Is your reason for being angry realistic? If you were angry because you didn't get what you were promised, then that is a realistic reason. However, if you're angry that you're not getting special consideration, this is not realistic.

Another aspect of realistic anger is the important distinction between the fact that people do stupid things and that they do the stupid things *to you*. For instance, you have a right to be angry with a noisy neighbor, but if you take it personally the result is a great deal of resentment. You want to say, "How could he do that stupid thing?" (Realistic and appropriate) not, "How could he do that stupid thing to me?"

It is amazing the difference it makes to not take things personally. I can remember saying to my friend that I hated it when people attacked me. My energy about the situation completely shifted when my friend reminded me that people weren't attacking me. They were yelling. I was able to recognize that I got angry when people yelled. It was unacceptable to me. The whole experience shifted for me in a moment. It became their issue instead of my problem to solve. It wasn't from a position of "It's your problem!!!" it was from a place of "How is that for you?" I had compassion and concern with no responsibility or ownership.

The fourth step is to deal with anger realistically. Obviously, a direct expression of anger is not always the best solution. When you know who has made you angry, why you're angry, and that the anger has a reasonable cause, then a frank discussion with the person may resolve the problem. However, anger is more difficult to address when the cause is not realistic. The basic problem is within you, which may require effort and patience to solve. Often, the other person is also dealing with problems within him or herself.

Resolve these situations by improving communication. Coworkers who take the time to understand each other's perspectives will ease the tension between them.

As with any skill, the four steps in processing anger are easier said than done. Stay in touch with the fact that people only make changes when it is too difficult to keep doing the same thing. Times of crisis bring the most growth.

I'm reminded of a metaphor I heard recently about transforming our experiences. Just like a bird in flight, we need some current of air to take off. Then we need just the right amount of movement and turbulence to grow. Your anger can be the impetus to lift off. Working to understand your anger will keep the right amount of movement and turbulence to grow and prevent it from working against you.

By challenging your anger, you challenge your filter and move beyond your personal restraints. When you surpass your self-imposed fetters, you will be able to communicate and listen more effectively.

Clearing away our blocks in our filters allows us to hear information clearly. Spending time immersed in something helps. The truth is that all people can be fine communicators if they are willing to be open to learning something new.

As a nurse you must hear the information about your patient, understand what the patient facts and figures mean, and make a judgment about how to respond. You are bombarded with masses of details and must pick up on the significant points just as the dancer must find the beat of the music.

When you take a pulse, you don't start counting at the first beat. You wait and feel the quality and rhythm of the pulse before you start counting. In communicating with others, you must do the same. You hear in the report and pick up on what needs to be done and investigated further. If Mrs. Jones has refused treatment, you know this may reduce the chance of her going home, and you check with Mrs. Jones to see what is causing her resistance. You are constantly hearing information, taking the time to understand what it might mean, and making judgments about how to proceed. This is the music of the nurse's soul.

To have effective communication, understanding your personal approach to listening is crucial. Though we all have a natural or preferred approach to listening, we need to learn different approaches for specific situations. Sometimes our focus for listening is just to relax and enjoy the process. Other times we need to acquire knowledge, so we must concentrate and pay attention to details. Still other times we must make a decision and analyze information to choose among options.

Nursing Dance: Listening Styles

The environment affects us along with our purpose and motivation. Additionally, the appropriate response indicates that we are accurately getting the information. The personal listening profile from Inscape Publishing, a provider of instrument-based learning systems, identifies five approaches to listening: appreciative, empathic, comprehensive, discerning, and evaluative. Developing the ability to use all approaches is indispensable.

If you were at a lecture or listening to a patient share a story about warm feelings toward a child, you would want to have an appreciative approach to listening. Your focus would be on enjoying and relaxing. You'd be motivated solely to be entertained, inspired, laugh, and enjoy yourself. You would pay attention to the context and style of the presentation. Language and humor might be important along with the speaker making you feel good.

If a patient were sharing frustrations, empathic listening method would be most fitting. You would be supportive and listen to the feelings that are revealed, affording an opportunity for the expression of thoughts and feelings in a nonjudgmental environment. You would ask open-ended questions or remain silent with sincere caring and interest. You would resist any urge to impose your thoughts or give direction until well into the conversation. Allowing the individual to discover his or her own solutions wherever possible would be beneficial. You'd be acting as a sounding board rather than an air traffic controller.

When a situation demands a decision, you seek information, and that requires a comprehensive listening approach. When taking report, your focus would be on organizing and summarizing the information you are hearing; relating the new facts to personal experience and identifying how they relate to what you need to do; deciphering the rationale for the speaker's opinion; and listening for the main points and supporting ideas. During a discussion regarding a patient, you would elaborate on what had been said. You would ask appropriate questions for clarification, bring up related issues, and summarize what you heard. You may be preparing yourself to share this information with others.

During the process of learning about a new piece of equipment such as an IV pump, you want to exercise discernment to be sure to get all the information. As a discerning listener, you want to know the main details for use and focus on the presentation or conversation. Your motivation would be to sort out the details, decide what is important, and make sure nothing is missed. Taking notes, asking questions, eliminating distractions, concentrating, and repeating for confirmation are key components for discerning listening.

Many times, evaluating while listening is important. If you are part of the team evaluating a new safety needle, you need to make a decision. If you were not sure if the information given by the sales representative was true, you'd remain skeptical. In this situation, your motivation would be to relate what is being heard to your personal beliefs and experience. Questioning the sales person's motives and looking for supporting facts for what you are hearing would be in order. You might respond selectively, stop listening, or even mentally give the sales person advice at times.

No matter what kind of approach you take to listening, what you hear passes through your filter. Continuing to challenge your biases is always a worthwhile pursuit as is confirming the message you are hearing.

Effective listening and recognition of your filters allow you to be a better communicator. When you and your partner have your filters in check and are able to hear each other clearly, you can create a safe environment for your patients and a more enjoyable place to work. Whether you want to be a dancer or a nurse, you must hear the music or what is being communicated accurately before you can free yourself to have fun.

Questions to Explore

1. What is it that makes you feel stuck, tied up in knots, or frustrated?

2. Can you think of some reasons why a person is frustrated at you?

3. If you put yourself in the other person's shoes, what can you see from that perspective?

4. How have you handled situations like this in the past?

5. Why did you say and do what you did?

To receive your free gift worth $29 go to
http://www.SavetheFirstDanceforYou.com/relaxation.htm

VIII.

Free Yourself to Have Fun

I run on the road, long before I dance under the lights.
Muhammad Ali (1942-)

When my husband started bouncing to a lively, single-time swing music, I hopped right along. We jumped around in perfect harmony with the energetic beat. By the time we were finished, people were clapping and we were overflowing with exhilarating exhaustion. We were so jam-packed with the pulsating sound that we were throbbing, our hearts bouncing in our chests.

I couldn't remember having more fun. It was all so spontaneous and vivacious. We kept the foundational step, step, rock step of the swing and added the vigorous bobbing as our own special rendition. We saw a room of smiling faces, observers becoming part of the dance. In our mutual admiration moment, we took great pleasure in watching our comrades have fun. Fellow dancers form a little community that non-dancers don't even know exists.

Dancing without having fun is like walking in a rainstorm with your umbrella blown inside out. You have all the right equipment, but it's just not working for you. When two people enjoy dancing together, it's a pleasure to watch. I don't know anyone who doesn't want to take dance lessons after watching a fun dance exhibition. (Well, maybe some who just go along to dance lessons to please their partner.)

*How would your life be
if you made the choice to have fun and created the possibility
of being joyful about being what you want to be?*

Try on the thought that you can create a new experience and
have more fun if you just make the choice to do so. If a doctor
is yelling or you have a difficult patient, you can acknowledge
your limits and express your willingness to help where you can
as well as your dislike for what is happening. Happiness is a state
of mind, not a state of milieu.

A nurse manager shared with me that she drove to work
each day feeling tired. She felt as if she would explode if one
more person asked her to fix another problem. She saw herself
being the chief complaint department for physicians and staff.
Her goal was to fix all the issues. She thought she would then be
happy and successful. With coaching, she recognized that her
job was putting out fires and helping things run smoothly. In
fact, her job security came from having problems to solve. Once
she recognized she didn't have to fix everything to be successful, she created an opportunity to recognize her gift for solving
complex problems. Making a full commitment to the process of
solving the department issues rather than focusing on the end of
all the problems allowed her to find joy in her daily work.

Another nursing leader identified a need for a nursing leader
to be in the building after five, when most nursing leaders left,
and seven, when the night supervisors came in. She shared her
suggestion for rotating the two hours among the other leaders.
Since the other leaders and nurse executive didn't embrace her
suggestion, she worked late every night with an additional hour
trip home. She documented her activities and shared her results
with no response. Each night she'd fell into bed feeling overwhelmed and frustrated. It wasn't until she stopped covering the
hours that the solution to rotate was put into place. Though it

was hard to let go, rebalancing her work and home life created more time and space for fun at home and work.

Once you see your pattern, be open to doing something new. It is the resistance to your feelings and asking yourself what is underlying your resistance that will free you.

Nursing Dance: Try Something New

Have you ever seen someone do something you would like to do, then try to do it? It's very uplifting to watch people have fun. However, it takes a lot of hard work before a dancer or nurse can relax and start having fun. With so much to do and think about, it's hard to keep it all in focus. Once you can, you are free to have incredible fun.

One woman took dance lessons for many years, yet she remained stiff and unenthusiastic. She appeared to not have much fun and was actually painful to watch, even though she knew all the steps. My husband, the dance instructor, wanted me to make "Free Yourself to Have Fun," the first chapter of this book. He insists dancing is not worth the effort if it's not about fun.

Learning to dance taught me the necessity of having some level of expertise before you can relax enough to enjoy and free yourself to have fun. Initially, it is all about learning the steps, holding your dance frame, learning to follow the lead, and knowing the right dance when the music changes. Once we get all our underpinnings stabilized, we can be creative. Our flexibility increases as we let go and feel the music. We can liberate ourselves to be an expression of the music. Learning to dance is learning to be a musical interpreter, free from inhibitions.

Nursing Dance: **Free Yourself**

Do you know what prevents you from being free? I read a story about Mohini, a white tiger at the National Zoo in Washington, DC, that spent twelve years pacing back and forth in her twelve-by-twelve-foot cage. When a several-acre natural habitat was created for her with a mile of trees, a pond, and a variety of vegetation; the tiger immediately sought refuge in a corner of her terrain. She spent the rest of her life walking back and forth in a twelve-by-twelve-foot area.

The sad thing is that this doesn't just happen in the animal kingdom. Nurses as all human beings fence themselves into repeated patterns and never notice they're imprisoned by their psychological limitations. The reality is that we incarcerate ourselves because it is comfortable.

We reach the limits of our comfort zone and stop. Even when it is possible to move beyond our prison and move freely, we stay trapped. We create the outside world based on our internal beliefs. We have certain expectations about how others treat us and usually find enough evidence to support what we believe. Unbeknown to us, this happens because of the way we interact with others. We are "blind" to the whole process.

The good news is that each of us has the ability to transform this. We have the prospect of restoration in every moment. Sadly, human nature dictates that we are only provoked to change when our life feels too confining or isn't working for us. While it seems more compelling to change the outside world to alleviate our discomfort, I encourage you not to waste your time there. Surprisingly, one of the hardest things as nurses we need to do is to receive love. We are not going someplace; we are where we are.

Nursing Dance: Receive Love

Harville and Hunt's book, *Receiving Love,* describes how boundaries get set up. We are all born with openness and receptivity, but sooner or later, our parents or caretakers wound us. The wound occurs when a caretaker does not properly deal with our normal developmental needs and functions.

The wound comes in the form of abuse, neglect, or invasion of some aspect of our natural self. We then unknowingly split off from this part of our natural self and it becomes our "missing self." We see it as dangerous because our caretaker doesn't support it. As we continue to be wounded and split-off, our conscious self becomes smaller and smaller. This unconscious burden of rejected self grows heavier, causing a loss of access to these skills and resources.

With our emotional and behavioral alternatives reduced, we face life with a limited number of defensive reactions. We develop familiar defenses of control, self-absorption, and codependence to protect ourselves from further pain. We hold tightly onto what's left of ourselves to protect from more infringement.

We attempt to make the pain of rejection go away by denying the needs that originally caused our rejection and replacing them with defenses. We resist satisfying our needs in order not to stimulate the wound. The defense is used to keep the wound out of our consciousness and results in us feeling empty. We try to fill the barrenness with things that only add to our discontent because they aren't what we are really lacking. Our lives become filled with self-indulgence or self-denial. We grab onto food, drugs, work, parenting, gambling, spending, starvation, or other reward behaviors and engage in them in excess.

Everything we do reflexively shows a trace of self-hatred and self-rejection. We project the rejected part of ourselves onto others so we don't have to stay conscious of it. Our level of self-hatred dictates the amount of love we can receive. It is so painful to become aware of and love that part of ourselves that we reject love from the people who bring it to us. We may even reject our own attributes or gifts that others see and affirm. Whether the input from others is positive or negative, facing the pain of our loss of our denied or missing self is more than we can handle. It seems safer to block information about our missing selves than to become conscious of our pain. To receive love feels more dangerous than to be without it because we would have to become aware of the deep pain associated with our longing.

Just like Mohini, the white tiger, we stay restricted to a limited terrain and miss out on the joy of life we might experience just to feel we are safe. The steps to consciousness are available to all. Move out of your comfort zone, take the risk of finding real joy, and free yourself to have fun.

Start by experiencing the love that is universally available. This will fill your emptiness and relieve your fear in the way that no one and nothing else is capable of doing. Twelve-step programs all start with accepting powerlessness and believing that a power greater than ourselves can restore us to sanity. It saves people from a life of peril. With this awareness you can venture into the unknown world of owning your feelings. Like an African safari with a guide, this can be a journey filled with excitement.

You need a guide to walk in the wilderness of your soul or you will persist where it is comfortable, no matter how confining it is. Feelings come from within you and are triggered by people and situations. Accept all your feelings as temporary. They will pass. Begin to wonder about them instead of running from them. Don't allow them to define who you are.

Move past resistance and turn to the power that will restore you. Ask for relief from your suffering. Whether you think your feelings are positive or negative, keep moving and asking for healing and you shall receive the desires of your heart.

Start noticing what you do when you have uncomfortable feelings. These are your conditioned habitat, your created boundaries. These are self-effacing habits that you developed to keep yourself safe. Believe you can venture beyond them whenever you are ready and willing. You have the key available to you whenever you choose to unlock the door and be free.

Perhaps you overreact to situations because of childhood tapes, self-defeating beliefs, past failures, or hurts. You may not even realize that you are overreacting because you think it is a reasonable response to the other person's uncaring actions. Because it is true that the other person's behavior usually justified your anger or hurt, blame is easy.

However, you will never break the cycle of pain and blame if you look outside yourself for the solution. You have a choice to take responsibility for your feelings, ask for healing, or continue the cycle of doom you have created in the hope of avoiding your pain. You will continue to feel the negative force that would like you to stay there. In reality, fully feeling your pain is less distressing than avoiding it. The choice to heal is yours to make. Running from pain results in overdoing and addictive behavior.

If you find yourself constantly in a cycle of burnout, stop and reflect on what is driving you. Anger, fear, and sadness are signs that healing may be needed. Honor what you truly want and clear the blocks you're carrying, and you will begin to interact with the outside world through your authentic power. Power comes from clarity.

When you are willing to be totally transparent about what you want and to recognize old resentments you harbor, you will be able to access the power that heals all things. The solution is simple, yet difficult to achieve until you accept your powerlessness, turn to the power that can heal all things, and take full accountability for your feelings and responses. Remember, the major issue people have is trying to control the things they cannot change. When you focus on changing others, you continue your cycle and never will solve your dilemma. Transformation is an individual experience that occurs within.

Nursing Dance: **Allow Yourself to Be Transformed**

Learn from the past, plan for the future, and live in the present moment. Be willing to be transformed. Recognize that no matter what transformation you are trying to achieve, challenges are inevitable. Strive for and celebrate progress rather than perfection. It's not only about the end result. Sometimes, people believe that achieving their goal should be the reward. If the end result is your only reward, you will miss out on many opportunities to celebrate yourself.

Achieving a goal requires planning. It necessitates breaking down tasks into manageable steps and setting up daily and weekly benchmarks to check your progress. Find a friend who will celebrate with you. When my son was young, we always had some kind of chart where stars were given for success. We celebrated after milestones were attained. At the beginning of a goal, we celebrated small successes. In time, more achievement was required for celebration. You can do something similar for yourself.

Find people who support, encourage, and hold you accountable for your action steps. Ask someone who has already had success at what you want to achieve and set up check-in times with him or her. Become each other's cheerleaders; it takes lots of energy to make changes. Most of the exertion is in the early stages of adjustment. Reduce, limit, or eliminate contact with people who drain you. You can transform any area of your life by focusing on it.

To reverse self-defeating patterns, you must turn the blame cycle into a fame cycle. The people you struggle with are the people who make you strong. Give them credit. Be thankful for them, because they provoke the drive to transform and the opportunity to develop character. Anyone can do the right thing when it's easy. Real champions persist when times are tough. The process of healing allows you to recognize the feelings and pain caused by past issues. You can learn or you can burn from whatever happened to you.

My mother was my first image of a nurse. As a child, I didn't have much of a relationship with her. As an adult, I came to realize that I had buried my deep desire to have that relationship. I created this same pattern in my adult relationships unwittingly. I never knew a truly intimate relationship and I was unknowingly afraid to develop one. It became my prison until I was able to see that my dream to become a good mother, wife, nurse, and helper came from that struggle. I didn't consciously know what was missing, but I knew I wanted something better. I am finally able to honor her with my work. My freedom came from the wonderful gift of forgiveness. There is nothing wrong. You are just the way you are and so is everyone else. Let go of the need to fix, shape, or cajole, and just be open to accept. We think things are good or bad, right or wrong, justified or unjustified, but they just are what they are. Forgiveness can set you free.

Nursing Dance: **Forgive Yourself**

Forgiveness is an important part of getting out of our prison. C. S. Lewis said, "We all agree that forgiveness is a beautiful idea until we have to practice it!" There is a difference between intellectual forgiveness and real forgiveness. Many of us think we have forgiven, but we have actually just disconnected from our pain. We couldn't have what we wanted, so we stopped wanting it. That part of us died and became our missing self. Feeling compassion for others' limitations, we became complacent and established a belief system that incorporated the fact that we couldn't and wouldn't have our wishes met. We continued to have a deep, unhealed hurt.

I felt sorry for my mother. She didn't have a great childhood, and her relationship with my dad was no better. I was long into adulthood before I realized I wanted to be loved by her. I experienced deep grief within me because she was unable to give me the love I wanted. For most of my life I didn't even recognize that I wanted anything from her. My disconnection from this awareness separated me from my deep longing for love. I had no knowledge that deep, loving relationships were even possible. I was only able to tell people what they should and shouldn't do so that I could avoid being hurt. I had no idea that I unconsciously wanted an authentic relationship. I didn't know enough to imagine what that was, and yet I held a deep resentment that I couldn't get what I wanted.

This may sound ridiculous. How can you be resentful about not having something you don't know you want? All I can tell you is that somewhere deep inside, you know what you want. Once I was able to bring this struggle to my consciousness, I was able to see how I was sending mixed messages unconsciously: "I want you to love me and I know you won't or can't."

We must acknowledge how much it hurts so that we can truly forgive and let go. Because unknown pain can be buried so deep that we don't even know it's there, this step is hard. We keep busy so we don't feel it. We disapprove of the symptoms of our hurts and we try to suppress them. It's all we know how to do. No one around us can see this "unknown" pain, but neither can we. We keep a smile on our face and always look at the bright side of everything. Our smile may flatten as the masquerade gets harder and harder to maintain.

A Nurse's Story

I always saw the bright side of things. It didn't seem worthwhile to think negative thoughts. I couldn't change that my childhood was difficult and my father was an alcoholic, so why keep thinking about it? I had to work hard to complete the things I wanted to accomplish. I didn't have time to think about unhappy memories. I thought I should leave them in the past where they belonged.

It wasn't until I got sick that I realized that my life wasn't working. I wasn't doing the kind of work I really wanted to do. I wasn't in a relationship and I wanted to be in one. True, I didn't have respect for my father, but it never occurred to me that it had an effect on my relationship with men.

None of this seemed to be a problem until my life became unglued by my illness. I saw that all this was working against me and I didn't recognize it, because I was always trying to do what was right and good. I didn't know I was hurting because I was always so busy helping other hurting people. I had no time for me.

The most difficult aspect of our growth is to forgive ourselves for our own iniquities. We will continue in our denial long beyond what is reasonable because to leave this state means facing that we have hurt ourselves and others. Once you understand the need, ask for the forgiveness from the people you've hurt, forgive yourself, and STOP what you're doing. The longer you hold on to the fact that you have done something wrong, the longer you will continue the pain. Forgiving yourself frees you. It allows you to make another choice. Once again, it requires getting in touch with the pain you have caused others and experiencing what mercy is. Then you can continue to make every interaction different.

Sometimes our first awareness comes as a sense that something is missing from our life. Being totally honest is the only way out of this. Identify what you are benefiting by not being fully in touch with yourself. Many reasons may be working for you to stay "blind" to your pain. If you had an unsafe childhood, feelings weren't safe.

This situation occurred when no matter what happened within the family (argument, ill health, alcoholism, or personal tragedy), by next morning everything was cleaned up. A perfect meal was served, and then off you went to school in perfect-looking clothes. "We don't feel negative feelings" was the message; "Maintain the cover by denying your authentic self."

You have a perfect exterior with a denied inner psychological world. Your defense mechanism allows you to function like an android. Even though you are very capable and can accomplish much, a vague, distant feeling reminds you that something is lacking. You also learn to not talk about your feelings and not to trust yourself or others. You may do a lot of talking, but not with a sense of ownership. It takes a great sense of personal responsibility to stand for ourselves and say no to things we don't want to do.

Nursing Dance: **Learn to Say No**

If we are asked to stay for another shift and say yes but resent it, who is at fault? This kind of emotional dishonesty will destroy any relationship at work or home. And there isn't much possibility of fun if we are overwhelmed and angry. Being angry with the wrong people, keeping us from the real source, uses all our energy. When we don't ask honestly for what we want, we have very little chance of getting it.

In some instances, we get angry with ourselves when we're not willing to say and do what we want. This inner conflict can result in aggressiveness. Because we pride ourselves at being aware of others' needs, we resent when others don't do the same for us. We miss the opportunity to share our truth when we don't express our needs or say no appropriately.

People like to do things for us if we are clear about our desires and ask with a free heart, not in a demanding way. Learning to ask for what we want is a skill that needs to be developed.

Likewise, it is just as important to learn to say "no" graciously. Express your feelings of being honored that people have thought of you and just say no when you don't want to do something. If we don't, no one will know our limits. It would be easier if others were more reasonable about what they ask instead of requiring us to figure out what is best for us. Compulsive over doers and over givers struggle with this process. Each person must figure this out individually.

It goes back to noticing how you feel after you say yes. Are you momentarily happy while the person is thanking you, followed by feelings of anger with yourself? Are you unable to bring yourself to say no or change your mind?

You can't keep going like this. It will sap your energy, and no one else is going to figure out what you need. You have to start being your own best friend. You need refreshing and replenishing on a regular basis—and not after everyone else is taken care of, but as you take care of others. You need to learn how to give to yourself and receive from others. It starts with getting to know what you want and then asking for it.

Nursing Dance: **Ask for What You Want**

How open to receiving are you? Are you usually the person doing for others? The problem with receiving often comes from fear. Prior programming to deny our personal wants generates our fears. Surprisingly, it's a fear of feeling the pain of not getting what we want. These emotional roadblocks can be the result of our unwillingness to accept responsibility for whatever is happening to us. The compulsive people-pleaser experiences an extreme fear of rejection.

Maybe your childhood was difficult and you couldn't take the risk of asking for what you wanted. Maybe your role in the family was to make up for what your siblings weren't getting from your parents. Or, maybe you didn't receive nurturing from your parents, and it all seemed perfectly normal. Everything in our childhood seemed normal. Sometimes we recognized our parents weren't doing the right things, but deep within we believed the problem was we weren't worthy.

If we didn't receive the love we needed and we complained, we were labeled as too much trouble. So we concluded that we didn't deserve it. Our deep sense of unworthiness motivates everything we think we deserve in adulthood. We are not good enough. We are not worth it. Maybe if we work harder and harder, we'll become worthy. But our effort doesn't succeed.

How do you ask for what you want? Do you bury your feelings and erupt periodically when you've just had enough neglect or mistreatment? You must figure out how to start asking for what you want now, or you will continue to create the same environment you so desperately want to leave. The only way out is to stop being a victim now. Stop wishing other people would fix it. Cease hoping that they will change, and begin your own metamorphosis by learning to take responsibility for what is.

Nursing Dance: **Learn to Take Responsibility**

How much do you affirm? If you want other people to appreciate what you do, start appreciating yourself. Any admiration from others will never be enough until you appreciate and value yourself affectively. People who don't value themselves don't value others either. If you see yourself undervaluing others, you are doing it to yourself. This is a great opportunity for finger-pointing or freedom. You get to choose.

How do you keep the cycle going? Begin to watch your patterns. It's easy to connect with needy people who ask too much when you want to act as a victim. Observe what you do when you want to feel sorry for yourself. Maybe you are afraid of something and instead of being afraid; you pick a fight so you can feel victimized. Maybe you care for someone you really don't want to serve so you can say, "See how they take advantage of me." You may be unconsciously asking other people to somehow go inside you to discover what you desire. No one can do this work for you. Even if they did, you would resent it. The real issue is your willingness to take responsibility for this process yourself.

Are you open to seeing what is really happening? When I realized that I placed this expectation on others, I didn't want to acknowledge it. I didn't want to be responsible for the creation of a solution. I preferred denial. I especially didn't like admitting it to my husband. How could I say, "I blame you so I won't have to be honest with myself"? Why would I want to admit that I didn't want to do the hard work to figure myself out? It sounds so immature, so childish. If I was so infantile, I didn't want anybody else to know. It was much easier to blame others.

Who surrounds you? Since we usually surround ourselves with people who have our mirrored wounding, it appears to work to blame each other. And so the dance continues—each partner blaming the other and creating a dance pattern that both know so well. Marriage is a perfect representation of this interplay.

The shifts from being a victim to being responsible and accountable will breakdown the self-imposed prison. The result is freedom to be who you are. The fun of being real is so worth it. You can say yes to what you want to do and no to what you don't want to do. You have power. You know your truth. You have control within yourself and how you respond to the world.

So, the next time something makes you upset, don't look for what is annoying about the other person. Look for what needs to be healed within you. What are you really angry about? What hurts? What are you afraid of? Find the root of the problem and you will set yourself free. You will not have to put out fires constantly because you will not have ignited them. No one can upset you unless you have an unhealed wound. If you don't get to the core and own it, you will be putting these fires out all over the place. That path is exhausting and totally unproductive.

What are your roots? One nurse shared that she doesn't think much about her father whom she saw playing a martyr in his later years. He was an alcoholic while she was growing up. When he stopped drinking, he became totally committed to her mother's care. She found it too much to watch for any length of time. Her image of her dad was as either a drunk or a wimp. She hasn't been able to get into another relationship since her divorce.

Do you want deeper relationships? We are only able to be fully in a relationship with others when we are able to completely relate to ourselves. We all have the deep desire to be close to others. We want to honor our strength and vulnerability at the same time. This nurse will be able to overcome the problem with intimacy only when she is willing to be intimate with herself. She must admit to herself how her upbringing affected her.

Would you like to have a healthy marriage? We can only truly be married to someone else when we are married to ourselves. Until then, we will want the outside world to protect our inside world. In this way we hope people in our lives stop behaving as they do so we don't feel bad. If we don't like the way it feels, we try to control and manipulate them to stop. In reality, our feelings are a statement about our need to be valued, understood, and accepted.

How do you feel about others around you? When we unite our missing self, we accept our feelings and begin to understand what we want. We may have to start by recognizing what we don't want, because it is easier to see than what we do want. We may have to admit to ourselves that we are creating a world where we tell everyone else how to live while disregarding that we are not living our own lives fully.

Do you want to create a fulfilling environment? In health care, we are balancing autonomous practices among physicians, nurses, and other professionals. The more self-knowledge you have, the more successful you will be in your professional relationships. Open disclosure should only be done in manner that is appropriate for the situation. The work environment gives you plenty of opportunities to learn about yourself.

What kind of openness do you have with people? Sharing personal information is not always right and proper. If you have unfinished psychological work to do, then make sure you employ a counselor or coach so you won't burden your work situation. Preserving the professional atmosphere depends on it.

Do you know what is driving you? As nurses, we often want to make the world a better place. In reality, if we work on our personal lives, then the world will be a better place. Otherwise, we are living the life of our ego, striving to impress other people with how smart or together we are. Our ego allows us to believe that all our frustrations are about other people, so we try to get away from the people who ask too much from us.

The reality is that we can never get away from the expectations of others, but we can recognize that expectations are just wishes. Shifting from using the word "expectation" to "wish" allows us the choice to go along or to do something else we prefer.

How free are you? The prison is unlocked. Now walk beyond your imaginary boundary. You're restricted when you're not truthful with yourself. It doesn't matter what your history is; you can transform the present moment. Maybe you did grow up in a scary, un-nurturing world. You still have the capacity for so much more. You have the ability to get what you want if you know what it is and are willing to face what blocks you. Search for it, especially when it seems like someone else is taking it away from you. It's your pattern you are creating; own it.

Do you think you are free? Actually, this pursuit is not intellectual. This means going inside, owning your feelings, taking responsibility, and learning to accept yourself for who you are, warts and all. If someone stimulates negative feelings, be thankful. You have the opportunity to know and respond to yourself. You are **response-able**. Your response transforms by transforming your focus.

Nursing Dance:
Stay Focused on Your Own Response

Own all your emotions. If you give others responsibility for causing your feelings, you are also giving them your power. The only way to understand yourself is in relationship with others. When you dislike people, it is really about disliking the pattern they trigger within you when you interact. You can learn to understand what is being triggered and heal it by taking responsibility for the feelings.

How accountable are you? Great strength is needed to admit responsibility for your life and everything in it. There is wonderful potential. You keep your power. You can be optimistic about life and everyone in it. Working together well with others creates a common good. Your enthusiasm and your gifts are offered in your world. Most importantly, you have more fun.

How proficient are you? Being professional means being above pettiness. We always have the option to resolve our relationship issues at work, and many people do. The work world is changing. We have workplace requirements from the U.S. Occupational Safety and Health Administration to protect the innocent. Of course, it is necessary to protect the innocent. Still, the major issue with solely protecting the innocent is that we are not solving the underlying crisis.

How much anger do you see in the workplace and beyond? We are moving to a new level of consciousness, more accepting of anger and entitlement. My nursing students and some nurses exhibit this attitude. This aggression originates in our internal conflicts.

Our internal burning is for something totally outside of our conscious awareness. So we must identify, acknowledge, and ask for our wishes. Just because you ask for it doesn't mean that the other person will give it to you. Many of us can't hold on to our wishes very long before we give up.

The frustration that comes from wanting something and not getting it drives much workaholism and other addictions. Our culture encourages giving things instead of ourselves to our children. We show love through money and possessions, and this leads to confusion and frustration.

People desire deep relationships, but many of us never experience them. We are so out of touch with our ability to have deep relationships with anyone, even our spouses. Authenticity is the answer and is needed in every part of our lives. You can see what you are expecting by looking at what you are getting.

Nursing Dance: **Know Your Expectations**

What do you expect at your workplace? A work expectation profile from Inscape Publishing identifies an individual's rating of ten key expectations in the workplace: structure, diversity, recognition, autonomy, environment, expression, teamwork, stability, balance, and career growth. People differ on the levels they need in each areas, but all are needed to some extent.

On some level, all need structure or clear instructions regarding what to do, how to do it, and the resources available. People value new and different ideas about how to accomplish tasks. However, this can lead to conflict at times. Recognition is esteemed. Independence and the freedom to make decisions about how to do one's job are appreciated.

The level of social interaction, though it varies, is significant for people. The ability to express opinions and be authentic is fundamental. Having a collaborative environment is highly esteemed and commonly used to reach work objectives. People want some amount of job security and dependability. They desire that their personal and professional goals be seen as important to others. People want their career growth goals to be respected.

Do you ask for what you want at work? Are your requests met? These ten goals can fall into one of four categories. Both spoken and unspoken goals that are met result in satisfaction. Unspoken goals are more likely to fall in the unmet category. Spoken goals can also be unmet. Obviously, unmet needs must be examined. Sometimes, identifying and communicating unmet needs will lead to fulfillment. Other times, thinking about an adjustment to other activities will allow those needs to be satisfied. At some point, people must decide if they can live with the unmet needs. Taking action, even in the form of asking for our needs, frees us to enjoy life more.

Do you know what your work expectations are? How do your expectations affect your work? What do you do with your unmet needs? Research on expectations in the workplace has shown that employment relationships are strongly affected by expectations. Employers categorize establishing and sustaining a positive attitude as a top priority. As people begin a job, certain expectations about that position are made clear, such as salary, hours, and tasks to be performed. Others are simply assumed.

Expectations influence thoughts, feelings, behaviors, and attitudes. All of these can significantly impact how we relate to others, whether intentional or not. Our thoughts and feelings influence our behavior. Open dialogue between employer and employees helps to uncover the unspoken, unrecognized expectations that can result in negative attitudes and behaviors. Greater job loyalty is likely when expectations are clearly defined and well communicated.

How crucial is your pay? Everyone acknowledges the importance of compensation, and everyone differs on how much is enough. If salaries don't meet expectations, employees will eventually find another employer. When looking for a position, it is essential to assess the compensation package.

The workplace can be even worse if people continue working with unmet expectations and develop a negative attitude. The reputation of an organization depends on its people. A healthcare organization filled with disgruntled people is not pursued for care. Understanding and sharing our different expectations is important to create a committed workforce. We differ on the amount of information needed to do our jobs; the amount of variability we can accept; and types of recognition, level of autonomy, social interaction, and the physical demands required.

People differ on the amount of teamwork and stability they want and need. Expressing these differences is no easy task. However, it can and must be done to bring more joy to your life. Get to know your expectations and decide what to do about those that are unmet.

Nursing Dance: **Know What You Value**

Do you know what you value in life? When I was studying to be certified as a coach, identifying my values was one of my hardest tasks. My coach instructed me to picture what I would like. That flipped the switch for me. I didn't know what I valued because that information was in my "unknown" quadrant. I had spent my whole life doing things I thought needed to be done. It never occurred to me to ask myself what I desired.

How does your lack of awareness about your values drive you? Before my acknowledgement about my values I was driven to please others and stay out of trouble. I never minded standing up for my principles, but I didn't realize the toll it was taking. I was exhausted. I was always pushing through my fear, accomplishing much. However, living connected to my natural energy is so much better. I was always using some kind of objective ruler. Now I can balance between what others want and what I want. It's a wonderful feeling. I still move past my fears, but once I have identified my wishes, it's so much easier to create the life I want. The shift need not be monumental, but with a clear vision of where you're going, you'll know when to say no and not be distracted from your goal.

What is your purpose? When you discover a vision that really fits, you will be drawn to it like a magnet. It will be meaningful and help others. Even when you're tired, you will still want to keep on task to reach your preferred future when you take the time to know how it serves you to serve others. No one has to direct your choices when you are inspired.

Inspiration is more fun than perspiration. I had this unconscious game going on for my whole life. I would figure out what other people wanted, and I expected other people to figure out what I wanted. It makes sense given my family history, and it was a great prescription for craziness. Don't let people drive you crazy. Let them drive you to consciousness. This is the real prescription for joy. We work so very hard to get everyone else to understand us. We actually expect others to take care of our feelings and treat us the way we want to be treated.

How about taking the time to figure out you? If you spend time wondering what you are drawn to, you will live an inspired life. You need time to relax, refresh, and reflect. It is in the quiet times when we get inspiration. Wonderful things happen when we give ourselves the opportunity to reflect. Inspiration comes and transformation happens. Our enthusiasm comes from being touched, moved, and inspired. We are no longer doing just what we want. We are fulfilling a much bigger picture. We are doing our work in the world.

What does your work in the world look like? What would happen if every nurse saw him or herself doing their work in the world? Every morning, we would be thinking about our blessings and be inspired to make the world a better place. We would then take very good care of ourselves because we would be in touch with the sacredness of our ministry.

You can't do your work in the world if you burn yourself out. Taking time for yourself and slowing down enough to hear inspiration is doing things the easy way and produces great results. Accepting ourselves is relaxing and accommodating our response to others. It is not demanding that other people treat us a certain way because we don't want to feel what we perceive as negative feelings.

Do you want to feel joy and have more fun? A joyful life is inviting people into an authentic relationship and asking for our wishes. The fun comes when we're able to appreciate receiving our desire because we know it is a gift, not an obligation.

Many of us believe that our partners or significant others need to make up for all the pain and hurt from childhood. No matter how hard we try, we will never accomplish this. You can't make up for past hurts. All you can do is truly feel them, own them as yours, see how they drive you, and release them so you will be free to move beyond them. Figure out the story you have been telling yourself, and you can transform your life.

I recently heard a story about a man whose father didn't show love and affection. When he got married, he expected his wife to pay him back. She had to try to make him feel good about himself at all times. If she failed to tell him she appreciated his help, he did a good job, and everything in life was great, he felt hurt or ignored and lashed out in anger.

How similar is this to your life? We nurses frequently take on the role to give people what they didn't get in childhood. We are generally compassionate and want to make up for what has been missing in their lives. In this case, the woman had been a happy, easygoing person when she and her husband married, but soon became depressed, discouraged, and angry. She dreaded coming home from work at night and didn't look forward to weekends.

If people limp along in an unhappy state while their situation gradually gets worse, they will probably begin to see the effects in their physical bodies. So many nurses stay in bad situations at work or at home because they don't want to feel the rejection of taking a stand and asking for what they want. By the time they finally say something, they are so angry that people just get defensive and don't listen. If we were not so addicted to everyone's approval, we would be able to ask for what we want and really have a chance of getting it. People who cannot love and approve of themselves live in tremendous emotional pain. If you cannot approve of yourself, you will always be looking for someone else to fill the un-fillable void. Once you honor yourself and recognize you own your response, you free yourself to have fun.

Questions to Explore

1. How will you know that your life is working well for you?

2. If you knew you couldn't fail, what would you do?

3. Name five things that could make your life more fun?

4. What do you need to let go of to have more fun?

5. If a friend had your circumstances what would you recommend he or she do?

To receive your free gift worth $29 go to
http://www.SavetheFirstDanceforYou.com/relaxation.htm

IX.

Add Your Style

*God creates, I do not create. I assemble and I steal
everywhere to do it—from what I see, from what the
dancers can do, from what others do.*
George Balanchine (1904-1983)

Encircled by mirrors and filled with the Latin sound of
rumba, we moved into each other. With our knees slightly bent,
we took small steps to the side, receiving our weight on the
insides of our feet. Gradually, we rolled our feet until our weight
was on the outside, at the same time straightening our legs until
we felt ourselves sit on one hip. With our opposite knees slightly
bent, we closed our feet, receiving the weight on the inside of
our other feet. Simultaneously, we straightened our other legs
until we felt our selves sit on the other hip.

We replicated the same movement with our opposite feet to
complete the box step of rumba. All our hip action came from
our knee movements as we swiveled through the quick, quick,
and slow to the seductive flow of the music.

I raised my right arm up to match my partner's as we rotated
toward each other. My arm dropped down around the back of
my head and down the center of my body as I moved around
him. He grasped my left hand and we moved side-by-side as
our free arms moved out with soft hands, relaxed fingers, and a
slight lift of our pointer fingers. We moved into each other as he

guided me slowly around his body with my left arm stretched out. I moved around his waist with my right hand.

Watching our movements in the reflection, we examined their subtleties. We continued to move in, out, and around each other to the sound of the alluring, provocative music. Each step and arm movement was done to add our style.

After dancers learn all the steps and basics of the ballroom, they are ready to develop their own style. This free style is an inner expression of self in relation to the music. An instructor can't teach this. You move in ways that finally feel natural. You communicate with your dance through your freedom of expression, the way a dancer holds his or her posture and movements. Facial expressions add excitement and capture the undivided attention of the partner and audience. Each step and movement is done with poise and self-assuredness.

As experience grows, the dancer moves from mechanical to flowing motions. Each dancer has a unique interpretation of the music. The two dancers reflect the union of their differences to create a magnificent musical testimony. This moment can only happen when the dancers feel comfortable enough to release their inner eloquence. Not all dancers achieve this level of articulation. It takes years of practice and an inner connection with self and the music.

Dancers who excel bind with their passion. Awareness and desire allow a dancer to reach a state of brilliance. Responsiveness and expertise are qualities of the leaders in dance. Though every dancer is capable of full expression, not all choose it.

How would you life be
if you became authentic and valued the gift of being real
in every situation and with everyone?

We unknowingly go through our nursing career thinking we have to be a certain way to be acceptable. Then something happens that shows us some insight into who we really are. Knowing and valuing our gifts allow us to be clearer and share more of ourselves with the world. Sometimes, miracles happen.

An ICU nurse had a postoperative patient who had vascular surgery on a lower limb. The patient's wife was concerned because the patient's limb remained cold and discolored. As the wife voiced her concerns, the nurse felt a strong pull in her solar plexus and said, "We are not going to lose his leg after all he's been through." As she made this statement, she put her hands on his legs and had this strong sensation that all would be well. In the next few days, coloring returned to the patient's leg. His pulse became stronger and the temperature of his leg rose to normal. Within a week of this incident, the patient left the hospital with good circulation in his affected leg. The nurse recognized the magic of believing as a necessary part of her care from that point on.

A medical/surgical nurse was caring for a postoperative patient after bowel surgery. Twenty-four hours after he was transferred to her unit from ICU, his temperature increased to 104.8 degrees. His wife began to express her fear of losing him. As the nurses went into action, starting an IV and using ice to reduce the man's temperature, the nurse announced to the wife, "We are not going to lose him." Before discharge, the man told his wife he had wanted to give up, but the words of the nurse kept him confident that he would survive. He told his wife that it was the power of his nurse's belief that saved his life.

Your intention is powerful, so don't be afraid to set it and share it. How much freedom do you feel to express yourself? Nurses have the same opportunity to take what they are taught and add their style. Nurses who fully express their uniqueness are gems. They are leaders because they are open to their own full expression. Never stop growing and moving beyond your circumstance.

Nursing Dance: **Keep Moving**

Nurses who have achieved experience and knowledge and are fully aware of their skills and unique gifts exude confidence. They know they can handle whatever situation comes their way. They can overcome any circumstance because they have buoyancy. It doesn't mean that all will be perfect, but they will keep moving.

These nursing leaders are recognizable because they are the first to offer to help. Being a leader is not about a position. It is a state of mind, a state of being. It is the makeup of being present to your profession, your patients, and yourself. Peacefulness and joy arise from knowing, accepting, and being you. Once this understanding happens, nothing can shake your self-confidence. No one can disrupt your peace of mind. You become the eternal optimist. If this is not where you are right now, allow yourself to move to a higher level of awareness and expansion.

Transformation requires the knowledge of several important things. First, we must all recognize that we are really only transformed by our experience. We can read and understand information, but that doesn't alter our lives unless we have a personal experience that impacts us and motivates us. We can misuse our knowledge by telling everyone else what to do and how to do it. But the people around us won't alter their behavior until they experience something that transforms them.

Something from within draws us to transform. It is important to slow down and become conscious to notice what is happening to our inner world. When change starts in your life, release your anger, resistance, and old patterns of behavior. Look for where you're being directed to explore more of yourself. If you do feel angry and resistant when things start changing, just notice it without judgment. This will help you move through the process.

Allow yourself to flow through transformation. Feel your feelings of fear, anger, and sadness and own them. Don't look for people to blame for your feelings. Notice and stop directing your feelings toward the people around you. It is easier to find evidence and blame others than to face our own issues. However, it prolongs the process. You can't control what others think, say, or do, so accept it without fear of consequences. This doesn't mean you make choices to put yourself in harm's way. You always have choices within your control.

Nursing Dance:
Release Fear, Accept Lack of Control

Become aware of your style of behavior. Release fear and accept your lack of control. The compelling drive to tell other people what they should and shouldn't do is a fruitless attempt to prevent us from sensing what we perceive as negative feelings. Keep reminding yourself that all you have control over is your response to the events of life. The more you try to control, the more you give away your power. We all strive to make our world safe. When we talk about not trusting other people, it is really a statement about not trusting ourselves with those individuals.

One nurse believed that people actually chose a different perspective than hers just to undermine and frustrate her. It was difficult for her to recognize that people just thought differently. Once she was able to view these diverse viewpoints as a gift and a point of negotiation, she found her experience with other people more enriching than fearful.

Trust and safety are statements about our state of mind. The sense of safety originates in the belief that we can handle the situation at hand. Our response gives us power over what we can control—ourselves.

Maintain the belief that all things work together for good. Life's experiences build our character and show us who we are. Once you are comfortable just being, life is easier and more fun. The simple expression of you is your gift to the world. Give from your natural energy; don't force yourself to give what you think is expected of you.

Programming to please others can precipitate giving when our heart is not in it. We can be so caring about the needs of others that we place our own well-being in jeopardy. We need to learn when it is our time to do and when it is ours to leave it alone.

Each person is unique and is gifted with a distinct history and calling. You may be a nurse like many others, but no one is exactly like you. We are all distinct with a particular way of doing and thinking.

We often think of ourselves as insignificant in the whole scheme of things, but there is nothing inconsequential about any of us. The movie *It's a Wonderful Life* makes this point so beautifully. We matter, we are significant, and we are essential to creating our soul position in ways that will be totally fulfilling to us.

We often miss how our gifts and position are perfectly matched. Our role on this planet is considerable and without us the world would be altered. Our systems are interconnected.

Everything we do has an effect on those who coexist with us, whether we know them or not. We affect people, and they affect other people. The world would be completely changed without us and as we transform, we have a profound impact on the world around us.

We are entrusted with the guardianship of our own life. Therefore, we are responsible for our own care and feeding. We need to be accountable and take ownership of what happens to us. We would not let people dump garbage in our house, so why do we let people dump garbage in our minds? It's essential to carefully choose who we listen to. As the saying about computers goes, "garbage in, garbage out."

Watch what you read. Choose your friends wisely. Expose yourself to truth. The optimist creed begins with "Be so strong that nothing can disturb your peace of mind." You get strong by choosing wisely.

Social learning theory indicates that the likelihood for behavior to occur is a function of the expectancy that the behavior will lead to a particular reward along with the value of that reward. People's behavior is also a function of their locus of control.

People with an external locus of control believe that outcomes in their life are under the control of powerful others or are determined by fate, luck, or chance. People with an internal locus of control believe that outcomes are the direct result of their behavior.

Health locus of control is the degree to which individuals believe that their health is controlled by internal or external factors. Since it is true that internals appear more likely to engage in positive health and sick role behaviors, it is apparent that the health locus of control emphasizes the importance of the health educators in training patients to hold more internal beliefs. Thus, many health education programs emphasize patient responsibility and internal beliefs. When we define success in terms of growth, we will find fulfillment in the simple things of life.

Nursing Dance: Find Fulfillment

Our culture generally associates success with having material things. Actually, growth, transformation, and engaging the divine connection define success.

If you strive for things you may get them, but you will never feel totally fulfilled and happy from things. True joy and happiness comes from an integrated life. It doesn't matter what you have when you achieve peace with yourself. When you begin to understand what creates real joy, you will be able to help others find their own joy.

In *The Power of Now*, Eckhart Tolle suggests that a person can be anywhere at anytime in-joy-in him or her self. Enjoyment comes from truly understanding and living consistent with our individual nature. When you force yourself to be or do something that others want from you, little joy is experienced.

You may feel a temporary experience of satisfaction from the approval of others. However, long-lasting peace and joy comes from finding your authentic self and beginning to live honoring your gifts. You become a leader who can then replicate what you know. You must first take the time to transform yourself. With clear vision, you are able to develop goals for your future. Without total lucidity, you can still move forward with four faiths as your provision.

As you proceed with faith in your personal vision, faith in the people who support you, faith in yourself, and faith in God, you can overcome any obstacle the world sends you. As you become fully open with yourself, you find authentic relationships with others. You can begin to transform existing relationships and build new ones. Open, honest relationships make you able to feel your truth. Living your truth and being your true self is a gift that you give to yourself and offer to the world.

Expand your authentic relationships to create a core support system for yourself and others. This gift of authenticity should not be wasted because it is too valuable and rare. Growth and change can only be fully realized in an accountable, learning environment where people are truly genuine.

Leading others to be the best they can be is done by doing it yourself first. Realize we are always in process of becoming while being our best self. Our work is never done, for ours is a journey, not a destination. Each person has unique gifts that can be developed through support, encouragement, and accountability. It's essential to take full responsibility for our own growth. If our goal is to help others, we must remember that we lead most successfully by example. Most nurses enter our profession because we want to help others. Where we lose ourselves and interfere with true success is when we take care of everyone else and leave ourselves for last.

Helping is a wonderful gift nurses give to others. We can help through our strong skills of giving advice, counsel, and recommendations. Moving beyond sharing perspective to taking ownership of results eradicates our benefit. People who discover their own solutions are more likely to follow them. Personal encounters with our own reality draw us to change. When decisions and timing are interfered with, people feel manipulated and controlled, which leads to resistance. People often question an outsider's directives and ability to know what is best for them. Being curious and asking questions allow people to explore their inner world.

Nursing Dance: **Ask Good Questions**

The greatest form of helping is to ask good questions, thereby allowing people to identify what might improve their situation. Individuals sometimes need a boost, collaboration, comfort, and relief. It's wonderful to help others with charity, donations, and gifts in times of need. However, when people are vested in the things they create and work for, this includes intellectual property as well. Instinctively, people want to figure things out for themselves and we can assist in the exploration. People lose the opportunity to learn and grow when we tell instead of ask.

Telling prevents a transfer of responsibility. If we continually save others from their pain and suffering, they lose the opportunity to turn inward and develop their own strength.

My Story

While I was director of surgical services, my mentor said, "You don't believe in God. Let me tell you young lady, God lets things happen and you need to learn to do the same thing." I walked away puzzled. It has taken me many years to totally comprehend, much less do something about this. My unconscious goal had always been to help others and control any negative outcomes. I wanted to see everyone happy and safe. I was driven to distraction on a mission I could never achieve with all the best intentions. I had to remember that people turn to God when they have nowhere else to turn. Though it was difficult to see at first, my mentor had given me the greatest gift of life. She gave the gift to see what might be possible if I would let go of what was. As I explored and experienced my drive to play God, I was able to recognize my limitations. I felt peaceful about how just being who I was made to be was so much more satisfying and freeing. She gave me her gift of perspective when she taught me to just let go.

Learn to let things happen! The most loving thing we can do is encourage people while they figure things out for themselves. If it's our children, let them make age-appropriate decisions. Our partners need to find their own way and then share it with us. They don't need us to point and direct. We walk together, asking for what we want and rejoicing when we receive it. When we don't get what we want, we have the opportunity to grow through that reality.

People who have an external locus of control and believe life is always giving them a bad time don't change their minds if we don't encourage them otherwise. However, if you step in to make things better, you're unlikely to succeed and you have failed to give them the opening to experience their own success.

Prayer is the most powerful gift of all. It transforms and provides an opportunity to see real miracles occur. I visualize a switchboard with Lucille Ball as the operator with hundreds of lines in her hands, and lots of confusion. She'd be plugging callers into the wrong people. When we're doing for people rather than letting them do for themselves, it's like getting plugged into the wrong call. We are called to expand ourselves and share what we've learned with others. That is what makes us the helping profession.

An earlier chapter described certain behaviors observable at work. Some behaviors are learned while others are the result of natural tendencies. Get to know your real character so you will be able to identify those behaviors you acquired as a means of protection. We all have natural gifts that direct our behaviors and we also develop certain behaviors as defenses, resulting from our wounds experienced in the process of maturation.

Our defenses override our natural tendencies as a way to protect us from perceived harm. Over time, these defenses separate us from our authentic self and our connection with our natural energy source. Defenses are developed because we have a belief that we are not safe. This belief propagates certain behavior. When we continue to defend ourselves from what we believe is unsafe instead of experiencing our innate energy source, we exhaust our resources. On the other hand, when we interact with the world from our inherent gifts, we are energized in the process. We each have been given a special way of looking at and interacting with the world naturally. Our gift to the world is to share our perspective from our unique viewpoint and soul position.

Nursing Dance: **Know Your Soul Position**

We each have unique roles in life that empower us to make a significant contribution. Soul position is the position you hold in life. You hold the position in your hospital as staff nurse, head nurse, nurse manager, clinical coordinator, director, vice president, or whatever term your organization uses.

Your soul position is your unique dwelling place. It is yours to discover, interpret, and define. No experience is ever wasted. You can use all your knowledge and skills to accomplish great things. We often get the positions we have because we strive to make an impact on the situations in which we find ourselves. We may want to avoid conflict or change the environment so it will be a safer place. We do many things unconsciously unless we are proactive about finding our motivation.

To bring consciousness or light to our darkness, we have to step back and explore what drives us and motivates us. It is surprising to find our stimulus is often fear. We will always have lots to learn about ourselves. Recognize that we will perpetually peel away layers and shadows as we discover our soul position.

Our soul position is our core that is connected with the divine planner of the universe. As you strive to realize your soul position, you discover why you are here at this time and in this place.

Bruce Wilkinson has written a wonderful book, *The Dream Giver* in which he describes the journey that a "Nobody" named "Ordinary" travels to become a "Somebody." He describes how Ordinary saw a sign that read: "Leaving the Comfort Zone of Familiar" as he was "Entering Border Land." As Ordinary continued his expedition he felt his terror. This was followed by the encouragement of the "Dream Giver" to carry on finding his "Big Dream." The story is delightful and affirming. It points out that if we can dream something, we can achieve it. Even though the path is frightening at times, it is all worth it and starts with leaving our comfort zone.

Our journey to explore and discover our soul position is like an excursion. Sometimes, it feels like driving through fog; we

don't always have clear vision. During unclear times, it is important to move slowly and attentively, while staying focused on
what is visible. I can remember driving with my dad one night
in a significant fog. He pointed out the markers along the road.
The white lines guided us around the turns. We watched for the
red lights of the cars in front of us and the white lights of the cars
behind us. He taught me that putting our high beams actually
reduces visibility. We moved slowly until we reached our destination. The fog eventually lifted as it always does.

We can use this same awareness when driving in the fog of
life. Don't stay focused on the fog. Maintain vigilant attention
on landmarks that you know and can see. Don't intensify your
illumination. Stay calm.

The fog is our monotonous worry. In the words of Charles
Swindoll, "Worry pulls tomorrow's cloud over today's sunshine."
Worries have been broken down into five categories. Forty percent will never happen, 30 percent we can't change, 12 percent
is just neediness, 10 percent are minor issues, and about 8 percent are legitimate. So we might say that 92 percent of what we
worry about is fog. We have a choice to focus on the fog of worry
or the facts that we know.

Are you willing to spend your whole life focused on something you can't do anything about when there is so much more
to embrace? Worry is fear, and too much of life is consumed
worrying about or defending us against what we can't do anything about. All we can do is make a plan and hope for the best.
We develop defenses to protect us. Getting to know and understand how we defend against our fears can be time-consuming
yet valuable.

Many of our defense mechanisms are based on the fog of
worry that prevents us from connecting with ourselves in meaningful ways. When we connect with our inner self, we are able to

stay focused on our inner connection and direction. This is the process of discovering our soul position.

Nursing Dance: How We Know Our Soul Position

Soul position also signifies where we are in our relationship with Our Creator at any given time. It is important to acknowledge that where we are is precisely right for us. It may be an opportunity to learn something. It may be an opening to help someone else. It may be an experience of pure joy with life as it is. We all want to feel that we belong where we are.

We want to have the sense of true purpose. We wish for a sense of fulfillment from our work both at home and in our workplace. Each of us must take on the primary task of connecting with our relationship with the divine and ourselves before we can have healthy relationships with others. In doing this, we become aware of our soul position.

Once we truly experience God's love, we are able to go into the nooks and crannies of our psyche. This love experience is fully accepting and open to transformation. Getting to know and love your character and your phantom self allows you to begin to trust yourself in any situation that arises. We all have a shadow side because of the defense mechanisms that effectively protected us at a time when we were unable to emotionally handle life as it was.

None of us escaped this shadow side totally, so we need to be open and honest with ourselves about how we have guarded ourselves in this way. We need to show love toward our inner child as it ventures out to greet us. It can surprise us with who we really are. We may have spent a career being confident and direct. We may find that we were protecting this very gentle, fragile, indecisive mind within us. As we directed everyone's actions, we felt that we would never have to face those fearful feelings deep in our psyche.

Becoming our own confidante and truly loving every aspect of our soul allows the vulnerable part of us to be exposed. This is the journey to self-love. We learn to love ourselves as we experience divine love. We recognize that we don't need to be perfect. In fact, we can never act perfect, yet we are perfect exactly the way we are. This is an irony that many of us find hard to grasp. When we can accept our perfect imperfection, we can see how it all works for our good and the good of the world. If we can feel our own vulnerability, we are more able to accept and help other vulnerable people. It is not our perfection that helps others; it is our ability to love imperfection.

When we work to love and accept ourselves, we are able to share more of the universal love that is available to us. As we get more in touch with our soul position, we can become proactive about our approach to life. Our soul position includes our gifts and our unique expression of goodness. We accomplish our soul's task in the world by being transparent to ourselves.

Fear of exposing ourselves is common. We hide our pain as well as our glory. We fear that we may be the only terrible one or have trepidation about the jealousy of others. It takes time to become fully comfortable and loving toward ourselves. When we experience Our Creator's love for us, we become aware of how lovable we truly are. When we love ourselves enough, we will be willing to share how wonderful we are with the people around us.

Give yourself time, space, and loving acknowledgement. The divine abundance of life is accessible to each of us. Our job is to help each other become open to it. At every turn on life's journey, it's important to know that your soul position is in the perfect position to approach the Divine. Our soul position is our essence and our point of connection. When we accept the affirming love of God for us, we know true security and fulfillment. We are more willing to being guided and make needed changes. We become aware of our resistant and negative emotions and how to release them.

As we come into contact with this supernatural love, we are filled with exhilaration. We share our vulnerability as we become conscious of our weakness and fragility. Because we are all wounded, we can have empathy for each other's struggles, even when we find each other quite irritating and confusing. Our bond with our essence is kind and loving, and it is our quest to find that part of us that is our true selves. Every opportunity can be used to help us uncover our true longing for expression and to free ourselves to do what we have always wanted to do. We are drawn to our calling rather than pushed in a certain direction from guilt or obligation.

As you determine your fundamental purpose for being, you touch your nucleus that is your soul positioned for greatness. When your inner core is connected with your Creator, you know the substance of your being. Every predicament you will find yourself in is an opportunity to learn about your inclination. Sometimes you are afraid of what you see and push away from the experience of yourself. If you turn to your Creator at these times, you will be informed of the loving regard for you. You are never a failure; you are a work in progress.

We all deserve dignity and prestige for our soul position. It really isn't a matter of whether we believe in God because God always believes in us. When we decide to turn to God, God is there. If we don't get what we are here for, it is only because it is not right for us right now. Sometimes it's timing; other times it's the wrong request. Having faith is what sustains us during times we are hesitant or unsure.

We must start living a life with a conscious declaration of noble extraction as our main destination. Our reputation and stature are temporary and our role in life need not be dependent on what others think, say, or do. Acknowledge your principles and live consistent with your beliefs and values.

No matter where you are positioned, there is equal distance in all direction. That makes your soul position central. Since you always have the advantage of learning and growing through everything, always choose in favor of positive expediency. Mastery comes from flowing with what life gives you rather than resisting. If we perceive the environment to be right for us, our ability to adapt will give us our greatest gratification and power. If we recognize we are in a place that is inconsistent with our values and we have attempted to make adjustments but failed, we may need to have the courage to move on.

Nursing Dance: **Learn to Accept Disappointment**

Our soul has a propensity for simplicity. Be methodical and systematic as you move through the obstacles of life, just as you would be driving on a foggy night. Learn to accept disappointment without collapsing and you will have the upper hand in everything you attempt. Many of life's circumstances have a way of disappointing us. If we can learn to accept and move through our trials, we can step beyond them.

If you can begin to lose without being defeated, you can dare to do just about anything and maintain a positive approach to life. Your soul position is your lofty perch from which you see the world. The higher your position, the better your vision will be. As you attach your internal wisdom with almighty wisdom, you become more in touch with your soul position. You're not just going someplace; you're already someplace important.

When you know your soul position, you're in the enviable position of self-awareness. This state is something that few attain and all should aspire to achieve. Your distinction and notability arises from your soul position. No one else is like you, so continue to ask yourself why you are here at this time and in this place.

Your soul position must be discovered so you can live consciously by design rather than default. You can then embark on each encounter, knowing your purpose with more persistence and determination. Would we ever give up if we understood we were heading for our true purpose and we believed we could not fail? Live your life aware that whatever you are doing, it is your soul's purpose in this moment. At times you may need to correct your course when you acknowledge you are on the wrong heading. Frequently, we need to assess how what we are doing will lead us to our higher goal of helping others.

A Nurse's Story

I can remember drawing antilogous blood for the Red Cross. I believed that my absolute purpose was to make everyone in my care feel special. I believed that I might be the only person who my patients spoke to that day, so for forty-five minutes they had my undivided attention. I felt that each patient was a blessing to me and that I was to be a blessing to him or her. It changed a mundane job into a reason for living.

Your soul position is your reason for being in the world. Nothing you do or say should be wasted. You decide where you are and your transportation to where you're going. Your contribution is immortal and memorable to the people around you. When you touch someone, you leave your indelible mark. Learn about yourself and honor your special offering you make just by being you. Don't underestimate your distinctiveness and prominence.

Your soul is positioned exactly where you are needed for a specific reason. How exciting is that? Your mission is to discover what and why that is. Your attributes and interpretation of the world are exactly what is needed. If you are experiencing healing, it will be the means of helping others. We are called to help each other. We are drawn to things that are our best way to help.

As we become more conscious, we can help others do the same. We have more responsibility as we increase our awareness. Through it all, at times we travel in the fog and other times we have great clarity. Staying grounded in and not deviating from truth will allow us to proceed with accuracy when our destination is not apparent. Recognize that sometimes we are drawn to one thing and while we're in route, we are redirected. Move through these times with the agility of knowing our foundation is the vocation of helping each other. As *The Message* shares, "He comes alongside us when we go through hard times, and before you know it, He brings us alongside someone else who is going through hard times so that we can be there for that person."

Is it not wonderful to think that whatever we are going through can help someone else? You always have a choice. Always look for options. People and situations are outside of our control and come and go. Our control comes from our response. Your soul position will never be something that is inconsistent with everything you are. The most elating experience is always within your grasp.

When we experience struggles, our soul is urging us to change position. It is time to learn and move to high ground in everything that happens. Our every emotion is a window into our soul. Our soul is always on a quest to grow and expand in consciousness. Know that when our fears and inhibitions are stimulated, it is our soul telling us that it is time for us to overcome them. Each time we master another adversity, our sphere of control is increased and we can navigate within a larger domain. The choice to restrict or free ourselves is ours as we ferret out our soul position.

Our soul has an affinity for confidence. It is our misinterpretations of life that creates fear. Our childhood fears are created when our psyche is not mature enough to deal with the things that occur. It's nature's way of protecting us. Our mind pushes the information down until our soul is positioned and our psyche is mature enough to reevaluate the situation from a more experienced perspective. The more cognizant we become, the more simple life becomes in the sense of how to overcome fear, indecision, and resistance. We grow more comfortable to continue forward when our path is not crystal clear. This is the time to walk in faith.

Be ready to reposition your soul with boldness when you see and know what you are here to accomplish. Take time to understand and fortify yourself when you are unsure. Continue forward expectantly when your course is not obvious. Relish the possibility of your own humanity. Make your inclination your destination and you will feel your strength and confidence grow.

Take the time to get to know your soul position. Begin to be aware of the connections between what you are struggling with and where your opportunity for growth is taking you. Ask questions. What do you need to understand about yourself? How can it help others? What are you learning and what are you going to do with what you learn? We can spend our whole lives spinning around the same obstacles of our life, or we can make a different choice and move through them.

You don't learn to dance without obstacles, and you don't become conscious without barriers to overcome. Just as the butterfly must work its way out of the cocoon to be strong enough to fly, you must work out of your own entrapment. We have all heard of the Greek word metamorphosis, which means transformation or change in shape.

Desire growth in a way that works for you, and release it at the same time. When we are holding on tightly, we crush the bloom. We must learn to have firm conviction about what we want and relax our grip on exactly what it might look like. This is why putting all things in the hands of the Divine is so powerful. This is the only effective way to acknowledge what we want and release our need to control the outcome. It can be even bigger and better than we think. But when we hold on too tightly, we crush the very thing we want. A fire is smothered if it has no air circulation, and a caterpillar can't become a butterfly unless it is willing to give up what it is. Just like "Ordinary" in *The Dream –Giver,* multiple dreams are given. We choose whether to do something with them. We have an opportunity to develop our character in the process.

Nursing Dance: **Develop Strength of Character**

We develop strength of character from our adversity. It is the meaningfulness of the struggle that makes it worthwhile. Viktor Frankl, imprisoned in the Nazi concentration camps, stated, "To live is to suffer; to survive is to find meaning in the suffering." The belief that we have a purpose and we can learn from our struggle helps us continue our path. The hope that we can help others with the knowledge we glean keeps us striving for more. It makes the struggle worth our while and takes us to a higher soul position.

A Nurse's Story

Someone once told me I would be OK in life because I had moxie. What they were saying is that I had courage combined with inventiveness. It felt good to be recognized in this way, even though I didn't understand it at the time. Courage comes from within. It comes from pushing through difficulties. Unfortunately, I went to other people when I didn't feel my internal moxie.

I eventually figured out that I was always going to be all over the map if I kept expecting other people to help me feel better about myself. It wasn't until I went to the source of all strength that I was rewarded with the people who would support me. I was programmed early to search for people's approval, and the end result was that no one and nothing was ever enough. Other people are sometimes exactly what I need, but not always.

When you feel the moxie in your soul, you feel the spark of the true you. Let it shine through you for all to see. Honor your soul position, and you give others permission to honor their own soul position. We are all on the journey and we are all afraid to expose who we are. Remember that self-actualized people want a closer connection with their Creator. It seems that as people become more conscious, they become more aware of the wonderful power of God that we have at our disposal.

If we will stop trying to control everyone and everything and step back and wonder, we can get a glimpse of what is really happening behind the scenes. We often get so caught up in what is happening in everyday life that we don't notice the opportunity to heal. As The Message states, "Listen for God's voice in everything you do, everywhere you go; he's the one who will keep you on track."

In a recent coaching conversation, a nurse shared that she was in a new relationship. She wanted her boyfriend to come to her birthday party/girls night out. His brother was having a birthday party on the same night. She was struggling to get him to put her plans before his brother. As she began to work through the process, she realized that she was trying to control her boyfriend to avoid her own disappointment.

We would rather have a major argument with someone than face the fact that not getting what we want is disappointing. It is disappointing to see something fail that we've worked on, to see someone hurt, to have our children not get something they want, and to not get something we want.

Often when something we don't want happens, we get angry and find someone to blame rather than feel our disappointment. We will do almost anything to prevent this dreaded feeling of disappointment. We might even try to prepare for the worst so we don't have to feel disappointed. This is the foundation of pessimism. In reality, if we will just accept that sometimes bad things do happen and we don't have to prepare for them, we can keep moving. Just as in dance, when you make a mistake in life, you keep moving.

Life gives us lots of opportunity to feel disappointed. If we can learn to face disappointments as a reality that must be addressed, we will not be compelled to control people, places, and things.

To add your style, you must take the time to learn about yourself. You can have a reputation for wisdom if you will live well, live wisely, and live humbly. As you increase your personal knowledge and learn about your gifts, values, and defenses, you will be more able to be authentic. You must recognize how you defend against negative feelings and learn to accept that life will not always deliver what you want when you want it. Eventually, your wisdom is something you share with others. When you know and accept yourself, you are ready to strut your stuff.

Questions to Explore

1. What gifts do you bring to nursing and the world?

2. How do you express your gifts in your personal and professional lives?

3. What do you want people to remember about an experience with you?

4. What can your current circumstance teach you about yourself?

5. If God were standing here today, what would you ask Him and what do you think He would answer?

To receive your free gift worth $29 go to
http://www.SavetheFirstDanceforYou.com/relaxation.htm

X.

Strut Your Stuff

Every day brings a chance for you to draw in a breath,
kick off your shoes, and dance.
Oprah Winfrey (1954-)

My black dress has a low-cut front, an even lower-cut back
and a free-flowing skirt. My husband, with his red sash around
his waist, and we are standing side-by-side on the stage in front
of a room full of people as the cha-cha music begins to fill the
air. Suddenly, he brings me into dance position and begins a hot,
saucy cha-cha. We turn, move side-by-side, and travel together
again. We move around each other as we enjoy the thrill of the
music in motion. We have rehearsed our choreographed routine
so we move with precise confidence. When the routine is complete, we are breathing heavy and smiling from ear to ear as the
audience breaks out in applause.

Our first showcase together is a success. We are both tired
yet exhilarated. We finally did it. All that practice and hard work
is behind us now and we get to enjoy the fruits of our labor,
experiencing the internal reward of knowing we did well and the
pleasure of the audience as they stand to recognize us. Our individual uniquenesses worked together to create something bigger
than either of us alone and more than just two individuals.

We were the manifestation of the music in dance. It takes
great faith and trust to strut your stuff in front of an audience.
Just before start time, a wave of fear and doubt had crept into
the moment.

How would your life be
if you harnessed the power of forgiveness and
knew you could forgive yourself and everyone around you?

Forgiveness is the process of letting go of the old and taking on something new. You can't change the past. You can put it in the past, or you can continue to regurgitate to no avail. If you keep doing what you're doing, you are destined to get the same results. Having the courage to release will set you free.

One nurse was overwhelmed with the need to please people in her life. She won the employee of the year award as well as awards in volunteer organizations. She would bake bread and cakes for her peers at work merely because people would say they were thinking about how good some of her goodies would taste. People at work would ask her if she was always as perky and happy at home. Secretly, she'd been depressed and on anti-depressants for over twenty years. She felt like two different people: the one the people at work saw and the one who was tired, confused, and driven to do things for others. She felt guilty and lazy if she wasn't constantly doing something. Resentment was building. When she uncovered the underlying source of her split, she realized she never received the approval from her parents that her sister did. She saw herself striving to get that approval from the people in her life. She eventually let go of her pain and hurt about the lack of affirmation she felt. This freed her to enjoy the rest and relaxation she craved so much.

Another nurse left her work environment because she couldn't get along with her manager. After a year in her new position, she felt the same way about that boss. She saw this same pattern of disappointment in other areas of her life. She was divorced and no longer had a relationship with her sister. She wanted to make a different choice than leaving her job again. During coaching, she realized she was unable to tolerate anyone who thought differently. She saw this as a long-standing issue. Further, she identified that she thought people were stupid if they didn't think as she did. Once she surmised someone was stupid, she was unable to be around him or her. The ability to forgive herself for her flaws made it much easier to forgive and accept others' imperfections. Her fear of her condemning spirit was healed through a forgiving heart.

As we chip away at all the defenses and ways we protect ourselves, we get to see our real selves.

Nursing Dance: **Find the Angel Within**

Have you ever worked hard to prepare and then suddenly, when it is time to show what you can do, fear takes the front seat? It seems that no matter how significant, we are subject to outside forces. We all need to know who we are, what we want, and how we are going to get it. This is no easy feat. Michelangelo, the famous painter and sculptor, took three years to complete the massive, fourteen-foot-three-inch figure of David. When asked how he could create such a masterpiece, Michelangelo replied,

> I saw the angel in the marble and carved until I set him free… Which is contained within the marble shell, the sculptor's hand can only break the spell. To free the figures slumbering in the stone…The stone unthaw and cold becomes a living mould. The more the marble wastes, the more the statue grows.

We are Michelangelo and his statues. We must free the angel that is enclosed within our armor of defenses and personas. We have the opportunity to uncover who we really are among all our limiting mind-sets, set in the false hope of protecting ourselves. Once we have freed our true self and become aware of our self-imposed boundaries, we have the opportunity to express our authentic self. Our true self is honest, loving, and accepting. Until we explore our inner motivation, we will continue to live within our mask.

What we want to do is just as important as what we don't want to do. We can openly say yes and mean it. We can say no and feel in perfect peace and harmony with our inner world. This is the sense of integrity. We are firm on the inside because we know and honor ourselves. It becomes easy to be flexible on the outside because we can honor other people just as easily. We are sure about our convictions.

When we respect our limits, we appreciate the limits of others. We can no longer be taken advantage of. We have access to our source of joy and happiness and no longer try to be the source of this for others. We bring our gifts honestly to each situation. The people around us are welcome to partake of our offerings as we no longer are driven to give more than we choose or by the need to please. We are aware of our higher purpose and experience the delight of fulfilling it.

When we finished nursing school, the first few weeks on our new job told us we had learned enough, but still had much more to learn. We had enough expertise to follow the steps we'd been taught while continuing the process of growing more capable. Eventually, we were confident and comfortable enough to strut our stuff. When we try to get more in touch with whom we are and what we bring to our workplace, we must be willing to expose ourselves to a solo display of what we are made of. How else can we know for sure?

We must be brave and do things afraid at first. We must let go of our fear of failure or being hurt in order to move beyond. It's risky, trying something wonderful, because we might fail. However, the alternative of striving for nothing and succeeding is so much worse. When you go after something, even if you lose, you win.

Perseverance is what builds character. You must allow your-self to move through the stages of learning. Don't allow yourself to remain in denial in unconscious incompetence. The first step to transformation is admitting your desire to be transformed. Allow yourself to become conscious of your incompetence, and you have the great opportunity to expand your horizons and free the angel within.

A secondary wonder is that you also free up others to do the same. Conscious competence is needed when learning some-thing new or being reminded of something rote. Awakening something that was asleep moves you through your unconscious competence.

Allow yourself to question. Be free with asking who can help you. Ask what needs to be improved. Ask when, where, and why things need to be enhanced. Consider how things would be different and what should happen first. In this way you can master life's obstacles.

My Story:

When I saw my first professional dancing, I was unconscious about my incompetence. I didn't know my own incompetence until I tried to dance. I soon realized a tremendous amount of work is essential to make a skill look easy.

Once my lessons started, I became very conscious of my incompetence. I didn't have two left feet, but I had poor posture, difficulty keeping my knees bent, and holding my body in position. I wanted to lead rather than follow. My image of becoming like those two beautiful figures seemed farther off than I had wished. It was quite frustrating at first. However, my dream of success sustained and motivated me. My determination to be like those dancers kept me working until I arrived. Just the same, my dream of being like my "Nurse Jane," the ER nurse I so admired, kept me focused on becoming the nurse I saw in the mirror.

I kept feeling the music, developing my skills, and following my instructor's guidelines until I became conscious of my own ability and competence. I had the right steps, knew all the elements, and yet found it hard to make everything work together. The showcase that tickled my fancy, given by the professionals, was a fluid, flawlessly synchronized demonstration of unconscious competence. Their diligent practice allowed them to be in the moment because all the details were perfectly assimilated and the dance became an expression of their passion.

Many dancers master the technique, but without passion they are not much fun to watch. It doesn't draw you in when the dancers are not engaged and expressive. Similarly, the greatest wonder of nursing is our natural inclination to take care of others. This sometimes results in our own demise. Learn to save the first dance for you so you can become a scholar of your own soul. You must develop an understanding of how to take care of yourself or you will slowly but surely lose yourself in all the unending tasks.

Self-care means knowing who you are, what is comforting, and when you need it. You must identify your calling, values, and strengths as well as honor your limitations. Giving and receiving must go hand-in-hand, as must the process of taking care of yourself while taking care of others. To keep your passion alive, you may need to make some important changes. Your fire will go out if you are not stoking it. When was the last time you thought about who is taking care of you? If it's not your concern, it's not happening. What nurtures you? Do you take time to do it?

The future is predictable if you don't stop and take time to analyze these important questions. You need to put yourself first.

This practice is very difficult for just about everyone in the nursing profession. After all, nurses choose this vocation because they want to show love and compassion for others. Their energy is primarily outwardly directed. That reality makes them good nurses, but hurts them at the same time.

The joy of giving is wonderful unless you're on empty. There is always so much to do to help others, and most of us believe there will always be time for us when we get it all done. Or, even more interesting, we believe that if we take care of others, they will take care of us. When it doesn't happen, we become confused instead of seeing that it is predictable. If we don't respect and become clear about what we want, we can't ask for it. If we don't ask, no one gives back to us. Even though most nurses have developed an intuitive sense of what others need, this sense is not a universal gift. We are not drawn to bring nurturing people into our personal life because we are the ones who do all the care giving. We have defective receiving buttons. Even more problematic is that we are taking care of everyone else as a way to escape from feeling our own past hurts.

I was out walking one morning and passed a one-year-old child walking through a small garden. As I watched him move about on his shaky leg, I soon caught his eye. In response to my good morning, he said "WOW." Before I left, he said WOW three more times, and I wondered what life would be like if WOW was my favorite word. Looking for the WOW in everything I did would make life just a little better.

Robert Schuller often talks about living in the "WOW ZONE." When was the last time you felt WOW about your life? Do you believe you deserve a life of WOW? You need to believe it is possible before you will do what it takes to achieve a WOW life. Your choices create the experience. When you believe it and expect it, you will find opportunities everywhere. If you find yourself in a situation that doesn't give you the WOW feeling, it's time to become an explorer.

Explore the inner corners of your soul and identify where you've positioned yourself. Identify where you are and wonder about where you want to be. Resist any attempts at fixing others until you understand how you are creating disharmony. Ask God for strength, support, and wisdom. Release your suffering to Him. He is the source of all love, wisdom, and hope. Alone we are lost sheep. With God as our Shepherd, we can find our way.

As nurses, you are in charge of the hospital. You need to know your source of power. An acronym for POWER might be Presence, Optimism, Working together, Enthusiasm, and Recognition.

Nurse POWER: Be Present

Being aware of our dance before we begin to dance with others is essential. Ask yourself, "What needs to be done?" rather than "What should I do?" The first question asks for a much bigger picture than you can do individually. Recognize that there is more to it than just you.

We are either going to be part of the solution or part of the problem. Don't leave our profession. Let's fix it. Nurses have the perspective that is needed to solve the healthcare crisis. Part of the problem is that we have a disease-care system instead of a health-care system. We need to develop a health-care mind-set and help our patients do the same.

In his book, *Reinventing Medicine*, Larry Dossey shows abundant evidence of an intrinsic, positive effect when human beings pray. His response to questions of prayer and placebo effect:

> "The scientific evidence suggests overwhelmingly that the effects of prayer are not due entirely to placebo effect, but even if they were, what would it matter?" He continues: "The answer we give to the questions about prayer have the greatest importance

for our understanding of our place in the world, our relationship to the Absolute, the nature of human consciousness, our origins and destiny."

No matter what the setting, most people resort to prayer or meditation when all else fails. Ask for insight and give thanks for all that is. Take time to appreciate the simple beauty in life such as sunrises and sunsets, even when you're en route to the next event. Don't take for granted the people in your life, but be thankful for them as blessings. Acknowledge the blessings of your patients, family, and friends rather than seeing them as a burden or another task, even if they are difficult. The people around you change when you change.

You change when you no longer stay silent when you're not getting what you want, when you voice your desire for mutual respect, or when you no longer yell back when someone is out of control. You have a chance of correcting the situation when you identify what is going on inside of yourself, develop a workable plan to deal with a bad situation, and execute the plan with expectations of success. Healing takes time and can only happen with great perseverance and determination. We must continue to heal our patients, our profession, and ourselves.

It is an honor to be in the presence of someone who is healing. It is a magnificent reward for being a nurse. To continue experiencing the joy of nursing others back to health, get in touch with how honored you feel to be working with your patients and other professionals while you heal your own ills. Feel honored that they have entrusted their well-being to you. Your role is to learn and help others understand how to move to a state of wholeness. We all must stay focused on the quest to heal our minds, bodies, and souls.

Too often, patients get disoriented and lose hope when they are in the hospital. One senior citizen became confused after spending four weeks in the hospital. His stay was supposed to be four days. He was befuddled, shaky, and distraught. The healthcare professionals were suggesting that he go to a nursing home. An empowered nurse convinced him that he would be able to go home if he started walking. He did, and his wife got a hospital bed for the first floor of their home. He was a new man when he had a full night sleep in his own bed. His first shower was a grand event for him. It is amazing to see how the simple things in life give us great joy.

Believe in your patient's ability to heal. Have confidence in your own ability as well as our profession's ability to heal. Find out how your patients were before they came into the hospital so you can help them remember what they are capable of being. Give them hope. They need your confidence. Our whole system needs you to be your best self. Love your profession, love your patient, and start by loving yourself and creating a fuller life for yourself.

Nurse POWER: **Stay Optimistic**

Believe that something good will come out of everything. All things may not seem perfect to you, but that's just because you're not looking through the right lenses. When things aren't working well, use the opportunity to learn something new.

Optimists see what's possible; pessimists see what's missing.

Optimists see what's right; pessimists see what's wrong.

Optimists feel capable; pessimists feel powerless.

Optimists see blessings; pessimists see misfortunes.

The optimist isn't always right. Both may be right 50 percent of the time, but optimists enjoy life more and have much more fun. Maintain your belief that all things work for good and you will see those positive results.

Attitude plays a tremendous role in life. Consider this quote: "I am convinced that life is 10 percent what happens to me and

90 percent how I react to it. And so it is with you...we are in charge of our attitudes."

Attitude adds up to 100.

A = 1
T = 20
T = 20
I = 9
T = 20
U = 21
D = 4
E = 5
Total   100

The word attitude even adds up to 100. To demonstrate this, I put the word attitude vertically down the page, then put the number associated with it next to it. A is the first letter of the alphabet so 1 is next to it, T is the twentieth letter, and so on. So when you think of attitude, think that it is as much as 100 percent of your experience.

Optimists maintain a positive attitude no matter what the circumstance. They will find some way to get over, around, or through whatever is happening. Study optimism. It is a learned skill. Develop it.

Nurse POWER: **Work Together**

Let's face it. You cannot do it alone. We are social creatures. We experience life in relationship. We can only get to know ourselves through relationships, which give us our reference points and reason for reflection. Our relationships serve as mirrors. When things are not working well in our relationships, we can examine ourselves to see where we are blocking our own happiness and success. Otherwise, we will always be frustrated, wishing that other people would figure out what is wrong and fix it.

Or we want them to fix what they are doing so we don't have to experience our negative feelings. This is so very deceptive. We need to work on our own issues and be clear with the people around us. Ultimately, success comes from removing our own blocks. Because in nursing we must work with others, we must develop good communication and relationship skills. Since we will not know all the answers for our patients, we need case consultations with others who have different expertise.

Consulting with fellow physicians and healthcare professionals may be done formally or informally. Our patients deserve a multidiscipline approach. Discussions must be held regularly. Be your patient's advocate. Find specialists within nursing and other disciplines when appropriate. Get counsel from your fellow nurses. Be there for each other so you can be there for your patients. Never give up.

Give into your feelings and own them as your internal music. You will hear the external music more accurately when you clear your obstacles from your internal chatter. Don't act out negative feelings; honor them, learn from them, and heal old hurts. You can create a better world for yourself and for the people you live with, work with, and serve. Free yourself of old baggage that no longer works for you. Join forces with the people around you. Learn to accept, alter, and avoid what is not working for you.

Nurse POWER: Show Enthusiasm

Show enthusiasm in everything you do. Tap into your passion for your profession. Live with interest and eagerness in your daily activities. Norman Vincent Peale pointed out, "If you have zest and enthusiasm you attract zest and enthusiasm. Life does give back in kind."

People with this gift of enthusiasm carry a special kind of energy. They bring warmth and feeling to their relationships and vigor and sparkle to their activities. To practice enthusiasm, make others aware when you are excited about something. Throw yourself into all your activities. Be known for your eagerness, your curiosity, and your willingness to give it all. Proclaim your passions. Hold nothing back. Sing your heart out. Laugh and be merry. Proverbs tells us, "A merry heart does well like medicine." Hearty laughter is exercise for the body as well as the soul.

To maintain enthusiasm, we must do something that arouses our interest. As nurses must stay excited about the care we give. We must recognize that every encounter brings something new and different. That is what keeps us engaged and excited. You can continually expand what you bring to the dance of nursing and make each connection richer. You can achieve and maintain that mirror image of your partner and your uniqueness at the same time. Enjoy what you do and experience pleasure in everything and everyone around you. Your individual confidence allows you to perform the care patterns with your partners. You want to do the work to keep moving forward and overcome your weakness and obstacles.

Nurse POWER: Give Recognition

Recognition is the last of the areas to examine to experience your own power. Start by recognizing your gifts. Eliminate any name-calling. Begin to recognize we all are wounded. As adults, we find our counterpart, the person who will help us expose our wounds. If we take the opportunity to explore and acknowledge what this is telling us, we can grow and heal. You and your partner can explore all the dances of anger, sadness, fear, happiness, peace, and joy. As you recognize your gifts, you can be affirmed. Love your areas of wounding and pain. They make you real and vulnerable, just like every other person on the planet. When you love your vulnerability, you will not need everyone else to side-step it. Take responsibility for your behavior. The twelve-step movement and others teach that people must admit that they are moral failures. Paul acknowledged in *The Message*, "What I don't understand about myself is that I decide one way, but then I act another, doing things I absolutely despise…I decide to do well, but I don't really do it; I decide not to do badly, but then I do it anyway…" Can you relate to this struggle? We are all victims of the human condition so have compassion, but don't reduce the standard to strive for growth in all areas.

Recognition is honest evaluation of your assets and limitations. It's openly exploring when your strong points become a weakness. It's taking time to understand our natural gifts of perceiving, encouraging, teaching, administering, giving, serving, and being compassionate. It's examining your behavioral style, listening style, and natural tendencies. It's identifying areas of potential growth. All gifts have blocks and boundaries. You have the opportunity to ask God and trusted friends to reveal more and more about you. You can just notice what things you see in others to discover your disowned or denied parts of yourself. You may not be able to heal yourself fully, but you can go to the great physician. You have the ability to look directly at the unmanageable aspects of yourself. You are able to be humble and ask others to help you. You can also seek out those who you have injured and make amends.

Recognition is clarifying your limitations as well as rewarding and loving yourself. You have no control over anything outside of yourself. As the serenity prayer says, "God grant me the serenity to accept the things I cannot change, the courage to change the things I can, and the wisdom to know the difference." You are incapable of changing anything outside yourself—the weather, the past, or other people. You can work on submitting yourself to the process to transform you. You can influence others by changing yourself so that their destructive patterns no longer work on you. If you transform your way of dealing with them, they may be motivated to transform if their old ways no longer work. When you let go of others, you begin to get healthy. They may notice and envy your health. They may want some of what you have. It is important to seek wisdom to know the difference between what is you and what is not. The process is transformational.

Nursing Dance: How Transformation Happens

Along the way, you discover that transformation happens daily. It only takes a moment. It's like popping into a new experience. One instant you're confused and the next you get it. With the choice to be transformed comes negative feelings and resistance. Creating a supportive environment for transformation will help. Being in a community where people make a commitment to transformation helps. Remember, it takes lots of energy to overcome old habits. Too often, people blame the system or other people when they lose their power instead of looking for solutions.

Your main concern is how you experience a situation. We only have control over asking for what we want, being open to personal transformation, or leaving a situation. Many people leave situations without examining what their feelings are saying. Look at times when you're unhappy as an opportunity to learn something honestly about yourself and grow.

As you embrace the process of creating new possibilities, write down your goals and decide what kind of support, encouragement, and accountability you need. Then find a person who is capable of sharing in an authentic relationship to hold you to take action. This person may be someone you already know, or you may look for a new relationship. Many times a friend or peer who has accomplished what you want to achieve is the place to start. Consent to being trustworthy friends, meaning you will be open and honest about your lives. Agree to handle what is shared with each other with respect and discretion. You may also look for a professional coach to become your cheerleader. Commit to consistently taking the initiative in these relationships instead of waiting for the other to act. Vow to make your relationship positive, growth-oriented, and effective.

According to Jeanne Achterberg, author of *Woman as Healer:*

> Healing is a lifelong journey toward wholeness. It is remembering what has been forgotten about connection and unity and interdependence among all things living and nonliving. It is embracing what is most feared, opening what has been closed, and softening what has hardened into obstruction. It is entering into the transcendent, timeless moment where one experiences the divine. It is creativity and passion and love. It is seeking and expressing self in its fullness, its light and shadow, its male and female. Healing is learning to trust life.

Nursing Dance: Help Our Hospitals

Our hospitals are losing compassion and becoming places where the only touching that occurs is by machines. There are increased reports of accidents, and bureaucratic administration has led to a cold, uncaring environment. It is nurses who are licensed to touch. We must retain our valuable purpose. It would benefit our hospitals to leave behind the institutionalized thinking of conventional medicine and enter into a holistic view, where prayer and intention are routine and people are taught the principles of healing themselves.

Healthy living is difficult to attain and maintain and healing is very complex. One would be naive to think it could be summed up in a short book. However, clear paths allow people to begin the dance and achieve success in improved health. What the new end point will look like is not perfectly clear, but some components of the dance are essential. How would our healthcare environment look if our goal was healing rather than treatment?

Imagine an individual coming into the emergency room after an auto accident. All emergency issues are handled in a conventional way. Intravenous lines are started, bleeding controlled, radiological studies made, surgery performed if needed, and so on. Additionally, a prayer or meditation is said consciously to set the intention for all treatment to be given for the individual's highest good. Relaxation and self-hypnosis are taught to the patient if he or she is capable and not already knowledgeable. Calming music of each person's choice is played. Laughter is used to help the individual deal with all the procedures.

Once bleeding is controlled and all other life-threatening needs are addressed, a chiropractor or osteopath does a physical exam and reviews the radiological studies. Subtle realignments to the spine and other part of the body are addressed if needed. A non-force technique is used, which is an advanced skill for chiropractors. The focus of the hospital stay is on wholeness, education about the body, the injuries, and how the symptoms affect the individual on an emotional and spiritual level. Mental, physical, and spiritual healing skills are started in the hospital and continued after discharge.

To achieve this level of collaboration, physicians, nurses and other healthcare providers would increase their skills to include healing touch or other energy therapy and hypnotic suggestion. Medical schools would incorporate the osteopathic and chiropractic adjustment skill to their education, or chiropractors would be added to the healthcare team. Each healthcare professional would personally have formal training in complementary services as part of preliminary education.

Each person is gifted with internal wisdom that guides him or her to fulfilled purpose and meaning in life. When negative things such as illness, losing a job or ending a marriage happen, they are opportunities to face fears and take charge of one's life. This book is about raising consciousness of what works for each individual according to his or her gifts and calling. Life is a sacred dance for each person to experience. Every person has unique needs. It is imperative to shift to an internal world that allows us to value the people around us and ourselves. Transformation results in consciousness. Consciousness means people will question things they once accepted blindly. Walking through fear is hard, but tremendously rewarding. It takes time and patience. It takes loving oneself enough to start and it takes faith that the dance will be worth it.

The path to healing is acceptance of holism and awareness of the trinity of mind, body, and spirit. As our spirit heals, so will our minds and bodies. Herbert Benson described the association of better health and religious commitment, noting that across-the-board religious commitment brings psychological and physical health. Prayer researcher Dossey says that:

> Today the resistance to reawakening to our inner divinity, of recovering our soul, comes not only from religion, but from science as well. Both hold out the promise of salvation [one offering it in the form of God's redeeming generosity, the other in the form of scientific progress]. But both have stripped us of our omni consciousness [his word] and our soul, becoming dark allies in this morbid process.

Peace and joy abide in the union of mind, body, and soul. The price for ignoring soul is reflected in the mind and body. The struggle is great, but the rewards are even greater. Richard Carlson, author of *Don't Sweat the Small Stuff,* wrote: "The truth is, life is rarely exactly the way we want it to be, and other people often don't act as we would like them to…If you fight against the principles of life, you'll spend most of your life fighting battles."

Accepting life as it comes is the only practical way to live, yet it is very difficult in practice.

Louise Hayes believes that all DIS-EASE results from un-forgiveness. "Forgiveness" means giving up or letting go. When people can see that the person they need to forgive is also in pain, the process begins to be possible. Part of the process is accepting oneself as just what she or he is supposed to be. Self-approval and self-acceptance are the first major steps to greater health. Self-affirmations can help people get on the path. Self-nurturing behavior is vital to forgiving others.

The skills that can help improve health begin with being conscious of the spiritual self on a quest to recover our soul. Each thing we do for the body we do for the mind and the spirit and vice versa. The average person accepts this concept with difficulty.

Consciousness is achieved by seeing the divine in each human experience. Being conscious is staying in the moment and experiencing it to the fullest. A former client of mine shared the following anonymous quotation:

> *Remember that time waits for no one*
> *Yesterday is History*
> *Tomorrow is Mystery*
> *Today is a Gift -*
> *That's why it's called the*
> *"Present"*

We cannot change the past; it is over and done. We can't control or predict the future. This moment is a gift to be opened, explored, and experienced to the fullest. It is the only time that is real. By putting the past in the past, we have an opportunity to create a new future in this present moment. More often than not people waste the present moment, regretting the past or worrying about the future. Releasing the past, re-creating our future, and living in the present is vital to health and well-being. The complex system of the human being has many mysteries that we learn more and more about as we view it from a wide-reaching perspective.

Let us experience a new perspective and see human beings as comparable to the cells of the human body. Some make up the nervous system of the earthly body; others are reflective of hepatic systems; and so on. Each cell starts from one union somehow mysteriously knowing what role it will take in a particular organ, ever moving through a cycle of replicating and adapting. We can only begin to sense the interrelatedness of the body of mankind. Each system has a vital role in the survival of the whole. Likewise, each human being plays a vital role in the survival of our world as we know it. From this perspective, one senses how hurting another person is hurting oneself. Like an autoimmune disorder, the body fights off parts of itself as if it were a foreign body.

"Those of us who are strong and able in the faith need to step in and lend a hand to those who falter, and not just do what is most convenient for us. Strength is for service, not status. Each one of us needs to look after the good of the people around us, asking ourselves, "How can I help?" *The Message* is a great source of wisdom for finding a deeper meaning to our lives. Be encouraged to be present, be optimistic, work together, be enthusiastic, and recognize your gifts in everything you do as a nurse.

If we see ourselves as a universal body in which each individual act affects the whole, wouldn't we live very differently? As Americans, we thought we were so protected because of the large body of water separating us from other continents until 9-

11-2001. Things we do or fail to do affect generations to come, sometimes without our awareness. Much damage can be done before we realize the problem.

When people develop symptoms, it as an opportunity to determine what the symptom is telling them about the disease of their spirit. If it is a physical symptom, the body is the most conscious part of the being. Emotional symptoms can be handled in the same fashion. Meditation should be very specific and focus on asking our body what it is trying to tell about our spirit and where it is lacking. It should be focused on determining what kind of self-nurturing behavior is lacking on a soul level.

We are born with an unconscious connection to the divine. Many fear the shift to consciousness because of their human defenses and hang-ups. When we stop blaming and start accepting that being unconscious is part of the normal process of life from which we are called to move beyond, healing can begin. Consciousness and reconnecting with our true self is the dance that results from presence, optimism, working together, enthusiasm, and recognition.

There is no time frame, no specific blueprint, but there are steps for this dance. As a nurse, it starts by saving the first dance for you. We are not capable of aiding the transformation of anyone else until we have experienced transformation. When you learn to bend your knees and maintain your frame, you become inwardly firm and outwardly flexible. After learning the steps, you are able to know who's leading and who's following and truly connect with your partners. When you learn to hear the music clearly and accurately, you can free yourself to have fun. Discover that you are a unique interpretation of the music you hear. When you add your style and strut your stuff, you know your soul position and are fulfilling your specific calling to greatness. To heal and become conscious of the power you have access to, you will find joy in every activity you do. As you heal, you are able to share more of yourself with others. As nurses, you must heal yourself so you can truly help heal the world. Transformation and consciousness are the pursuit of health, wealth, and happiness, the hope for all mankind.

Questions to Explore

1. Who are you? Ask yourself this at least five times to dig deep into your essence.

2. Do you see patterns of behavior in your life? What are they? Where do they come out?

3. Are you striving to please others? Who are those people? Who do they represent?

4. Who are the people in your life you want to forgive? How can you let go of your hurts and see yourself as the source of the issue?

5. What do you need to forgive yourself for?

To receive your free gift worth $29 go to
http://www.SavetheFirstDanceforYou.com/relaxation.htm

Bibliography

Achterberg, Jeanne. *Woman as Healer*. Boston: Shambhala Publications, 1990.

Alcoholics Anonymous, (1976) Alcoholics Anonymous Worked Services, Inc., New York, NY.Brauer, A., Simons, A., 2000

Astin, John A. "Why patients use alternative medicine." *The Journal of the American Medical Association*, 279 (1996), 1548-1559.

Benson, Herbert. *The Relaxation Response*. New York: William Morrow and Company, 1975.

———. *Timeless Healing*. New York: Scribner, 1996.

———, and Eileen Stuart. *The Wellness Book, The Comprehensive Guide to Maintaining Health and Treating Stress-Related Illness*. New York: Birch Lane Press, 1992.

Borysenko, Joan. *Mending the Body, Mending the Mind*. New York: Bantam Books, 1987.

Brennan, Barbara Ann. *Light Emergence*. New York: Bantam Books, 1993.

Campbell, Don. *The Mozart Effect*. New York: Avon, 1997.

Carlson, Dwight. *Overcoming Hurts & Anger*. Eugene, OR: Harvest House Publishers, 1981.

Carlson, Richard. *Don't Sweat the Small Stuff*. New York: Hyperion, 1997.

Carnegie, Dale. *How to Stop Worrying and Start Living*. New York: Simon & Schuster, 1948.

Chopra, Deepak. *Ageless Body Timeless Mind*. New York: Harmony Books, 1993.

Cloud, Henry, and John Townsend. *Boundaries*. Grand Rapids, MI: Zondervan, 1992.

Cousins, Norman. *Anatomy of an Illness*. New York: W. W. Norton & Company, 1979.

Dossey, Larry. *Healing Words: The Power of Prayer and the Practice of Medicine*. San Francisco: HarperCollins, 1989.

———. *Recovery of the Soul: A Scientific and Spiritual Search*. New York: Bantam Books, 1989.

————. *Reinventing Medicine: Beyond Mind-Body to a New Era of Healing.* San Francisco: HarperCollins, 1999.

DiSC Profile. Minneapolis: Inscape Publishing.

Eldredge, John, and Stasi Eldredge. *Captivating.* Nashville, TN: Nelson Books, 2005.

Fortune, Don, and Katie Fortune. *Discover Your God Given Gifts.* Grand Rapids, MI: Chosen Books, 1987.

Fox, Matthew. *The Coming of the Cosmic Christ.* San Francisco: HarperCollins, 1940.

————. *Creation Spirituality.* San Francisco: HarperCollins, 1991.

————. *A Spirituality Named Compassion and the Healing of the Global Village, Humpty Dumpty and US.* San Francisco: Harper & Row, 1979.

Hay, Louise L. *You Can Heal Your Life.* Santa Monica, CA: Hay House, 1984.

Helpern, Stephen. "Music That Heals." *Venture Inward*, 14 (1998), 23-31.

Hendrix, Harville, and Helen Lakelly Hunt. Receiving Love. New York: Atria Books, 2004.

Kabat-Zinn, Jon. *Full Catastrophe Living.* New York: Dell Publishing, 1990.

————. *Wherever You Go, There You Are.* New York: Hyperion, 1994.

Logan, David, and John King. *The Coaching Revolution.* Holbrook, MA: Adams Media, 2001.

Madow, Leo. *Anger.* New York: Charles Scribner's Sons, 1972.

McGraw, Phillip C. *Self Matters.* New York: Simon & Schuster, 2001.

Meyer, Joyce. *Approval Addiction.* New York: Warner Faith, 2005.

Moore, Thomas. *Care of the Soul.* New York: Harper Perennial, 1994.

Myss, Carolyn. *Why People Don't Heal and How They Can.* New York: Harmony Books, 1997.

O'Murchu, Diarmuid. *Quantum Theology.* New York: Crossroad Publishing, 1998.

Ornish, Dean. *Love & Survival.* New York: HarperCollins, 1996.

Osteen, Joel. *Your Best Life Now.* New York: Warner Faith, 2004.

Peterson, Eugene H. *The Message.*

Phillips, Bob, and Kimberly Alyn. *How to Deal with Annoying People.* Eugene, OR: Harvest House Publishers, 2005.

Schuller, Robert H. *If You Can Dream It You Can Do It.* Garden Grove, CA: Crystal Cathedral Ministries, 2003.

————, and Robert A. Schuller. *How Under goers Become Over comers!* Garden Grove, CA: Crystal Cathedral Ministries, 2001.

Seligman, Martin. *Learned Optimism.* New York: Simon & Schuster,

Selye, Hans. *The Stress of Life.* New York: McGraw-Hill, 1976Y.

Tolle, Eckhart. *The Power of Now.* Novato, CA: New World Library, 1999.

Umidi, Joseph. *Transformational Coaching.* Virginia Beach, VA: Xulon Press, 2005.

Whitmore, John. *Coaching for Performance.* Yarmouth, ME: Nicholas Brealey Publishing, 2004.

Wilkinson, Bruce. *The Dream Giver.* Sisters, OR: Multnomah Publishers, 2003.